Nursing Ethics

Holistic Caring Practice

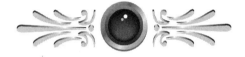

NURSING ETHICS
Holistic Caring Practice
Second Edition

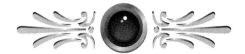

Anne H. Bishop
Professor of Nursing Emerita
Lynchburg College
Lynchburg, Virginia

John R. Scudder, Jr.
Professor of Philosophy Emeritus
Lynchburg College
Lynchburg, Virginia

JONES AND BARTLETT PUBLISHERS
Sudbury, Massachusetts
BOSTON   TORONTO   LONDON   SINGAPORE

World Headquarters
Jones and Bartlett Publishers
40 Tall Pine Drive
Sudbury, MA 01776
978-443-5000
www.jbpub.com
info@jbpub.com

Jones and Bartlett Publishers Canada
2406 Nikanna Road
Mississauga, Ontario
Canada L5C 2W6

Jones and Bartlett Publishers International
Barb House, Barb Mews
London W6 7PA
UK

ISBN: 0-7637-1426-7

Copyright © 2001 by Jones and Bartlett Publishers, Inc.

Library of Congress Cataloging-in-Publication Data
Bishop, Anne H., 1935-
　Nursing ethics: holistic caring practice / Anne H. Bishop, John R. Scudder, Jr.—2nd ed.
　　p.; cm.
　Includes bibliographical references and index.
　ISBN 0-7637-1426-7
　1. Nursing ethics. 2. Holistic nursing. I. Scudder, John R., 1926– II. Title.
　[DNLM: 1. Ethics, Nursing. 2. Holistic Nursing. 3. Philosophy, Nursing. WY 85 B613n 2001]
　RT85 .B57 2001
　174'.2—dc21
　　　　　　　　　　　　　　　　　　　　　　　　　　　　　　00-037113

All rights reserved. No part of the material protected by this copyright notice may be reproduced or utilized in any form, electronic or mechanical, including photocopying, recording, or any information storage or retrieval system, without written permission from the copyright owner.

Production Credits
Acquisitions Editor: John Danielowich
Production Editor: Rebecca S. Marks
Editorial/Production Assistant: Christine Tridente
Director of Manufacturing and Inventory Control: Therese Bräuer
Cover Design: AnneMarie Lemoine
Design and Composition: Carlisle Communications, Ltd.
Printing and Binding: Malloy Lithographing
Cover printing: Malloy Lithographing

Printed in the United States of America
04 03 02 01 00　　10 9 8 7 6 5 4 3 2 1

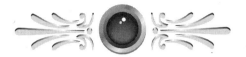

PREFACE

Richard Zaner, in his foreword to the first edition, gives a perceptive account of the development of health care ethics that sets the ethical context for this book. Although that development, and specifically Zaner's ethics, has contributed to our interpretation of nursing ethics, our treatment of the subject grew out of our phenomenological investigation of the meaning of nursing. From examining nursing as it is practiced, we interpreted nursing as the practice of caring. Because nursing, like all practices, has a dominant moral sense and caring itself is a moral activity, nursing ethics is inherent in nursing practice. Sara Fry, in her foreword to this edition, shows how our approach contributes to nursing ethics and to nursing.

Nursing ethics primarily concerns articulating the moral sense of nursing and appraising how it is fulfilled, rather than applying ethical theories to nursing practice. The moral sense of nursing is fulfilled through the caring presence of nurses that achieves the therapeutic intent of nursing practice. This interpretation of nursing practice requires that nursing ethics begin with and adhere to the moral sense of nursing. When the moral sense of nursing is realized, nursing ethics becomes engaged in nursing practice itself. The moral sense of practice, not ethical theory, is the driving force of nursing ethics.

We are grateful to many people for helping us develop and publish this book. Over the years we have shared works in progress with Richard Zaner and Patricia Benner for their critical appraisal and dialogical response. Zaner has long contributed to our interpretations of health care and of ethics. We owe to him the suggestion that we conclude the first edition with a dialogue concerning the meaning of nursing ethics as each of us has come to understand it. Benner, who has contributed substantially to our previous work, has applied her penetrating criticism and productive suggestions to the first edition. Sara Fry, over the years, has worked with us in projects related to ethics and the philosophy of nursing that have contributed to our attempt to interpret nursing philosophically.

In Robert Ginsberg, editor of the first edition, we found a kindred spirit who made suggestions that freed us from the stuffy language that plagues those of us who learned to write in the academy. His deep sensitivity to what we are doing encouraged us to be creative in tone and language, as well as in content. We are thankful that Clayton C. Jones and Greg Vis completed the project initiated by Arthur Bartlett so that our book will be available specifically to a nursing audience. The staff of Jones and Bartlett worked to get this second edition into print under unusual circumstances. We are especially thankful to John Danielowich, Christine Tridente, and Rebecca Marks for the cooperative and efficient way in which they contributed to the completion of this project.

For their encouragement, patience, and support during our many research and writing projects, we once again thank our spouses, Mary and Bobby.

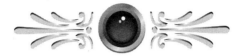

Foreword to First Edition

A little over thirty years ago, philosophers began to become directly involved with the health professions. Their efforts focused primarily on ethics, and these in turn almost exclusively concerned medicine: physicians, not nurses, were the focal point; the physician-patient relationship, not that between nurses and patients, held the limelight. Not surprisingly, within that focus, philosophers concerned with ethics tended to be more captivated by the publicly prominent topics of the day than by the actual practices of physicians; much of their agenda, as it were, was (and in many ways continues to be) set by the media. The table of contents of practically any "textbook" tells the story:[1] abortion, definition of death, organ transplantation, do-not-resuscitate orders, withdrawing and withholding life supports, living will, distributing scarce resources, human experimentation, and the like.

To learn about "ethics and health care" was to learn primarily about the sorts of problems that confronted physicians—and, of course, patients—for the most part in acute-care, *crisis* situations. Philosophers, of course, were not seen (perhaps with greater wisdom than was realized) as decision makers (decisions belong to doctors and patients); at best, philosophers could perform "ethical analyses" and perhaps make recommendations based upon them. Ethical analysis, furthermore, was mostly thought to be a matter of "applying" certain "principles" and "rules" (both taken as already at hand) to practical situations. But as there are many different ethical theories and principles at hand that are at odds with each other,[2] doctors reasonably asked "ethicists" which of the theories was the "right" one—a question at once decidedly uncomfortable (hardly settled within the hallowed halls of philosophy) and impossible to answer (presuming, as it does, a point of view enjoyed by no mere human).

For all the difficulties, nevertheless, one approach quickly won wide favor. With "human rights" increasingly endorsed, it was accepted that one particular principle was basic—a principle derived in substantial part from legal cases in the 1950s and 1960s, and from public discussions centered around questions of human experimentation (which highlighted such options as "informed consent" and "confidentiality"). This principle was *autonomy*, the "right of self-determination." On the other hand, it was also noted that physicians were by tradition, and often by inclination, guided by two principles apparently different from autonomy: helping patients—*beneficence*—and, if unable to help them, then doing them no harm—*nonmaleficence*. The real question, then, was how to balance the patient's autonomy with the doctor's responsibility short of falling into a kind of relativism or even anarchy (where too much autonomy leads), or on the other hand into an unfortunate arrogance (paternalism that results from too much stress on the doctor's beneficence). Since medical care in our times requires equitable management of scarce resources, *justice* also came to play a prominent role.[3] The work of ethics thus came to mean little more than applying these principles to the facts of any case.[4]

If anything, nurses were, like social workers and other health professionals, left to their own devices—including attending to questions of ethics. Even here, however, learning about ethics most often meant encountering the same ideas found in the bulk of the ethics (not inaccurately termed "medical ethics") literature: autonomy, beneficence, nonmaleficence, justice. If a nurse wanted to know about ethics, the thing to do was to ask the "expert," a person well-schooled in ethics—which commonly meant a philosopher who, of course, pretty much advocated the same line as was already well accepted. What passed for "nursing ethics" thus differed but slightly from "medical ethics"—despite the fact that most nurses had considerable difficulty seeing themselves as in the midst of "ethical issues" only when in a "crisis" of the sort found in the burgeoning ethics literature. Both "medical" and "nursing" ethics, as well as the ethics governing other health professionals (and, presumably, patients and families, though these were only rarely analyzed as such[5]) were thus regarded as a matter of the application of ethical theories already on hand—one in particular taking precedence: autonomy. Philosophers analyzed, physicians applied. Nurses and the other health professionals for the most part looked on, according to what critical action was taking place, and where.

This view of nursing began to be challenged from within nursing itself, with Sally Gadow (also a philosopher),[6] Patricia Benner,[7] and Bishop and Scudder (the latter a philosopher)[8][9] leading the way and basing much of their thinking on and in response to the feminist ethics of Nell Noddings[10] and Carol Gilligan.[11] They brought quite a "different voice" to bear on questions of ethics and health care, especially regarding the role of nurses in caring for patients. They, and growing numbers of other nurses (and a few philosophers), exhibited not only a well-honed critical discontent with the accepted "principlist" view,[12] but also a keen sense that developing a sound idea of *nursing* ethics requires being specially attentive and responsive to the particularities and circumstances of actual nursing practices (an insight that other writers on ethics were bringing to bear on medicine as well[13]).

The several writings by Anne Bishop and Jack Scudder have been at the forefront of both the criticism and the attention to nursing and to the "ethics" that is firmly and integrally embedded in its practices. In their earlier works, they were not, however, specifically concerned with developing that "ethics," believing that they needed, first of all, to be as clear as possible about the nature and character of nursing practice. Nurses, perhaps uniquely, practice "in-between" patients and doctors, patients and family members, chaplains and doctors, often in between nurses and doctors and even doctors and doctors. At the same time, their practice brings them in direct, wholly intimate contact with patients—the subjects of their most immediate concern—through touching, talking, feeling, and listening. Nurses' actions are designed to comfort, ease, calm, encourage, and assist in order to, as Bishop and Scudder insist in the present study, "foster the well-being of others" (p. 9). In this "way of being [that] fosters trust, mutual concern, and positive attitudes that promote good health" (p. 41), is a key insight that guides their approach to the ethics of nursing: it is a profession, to be sure, but here the "profession does not establish the moral sense. The moral sense establishes the profession" (p. 79)—a point that could well be made about any of the health professions. In their new work, there is not only a continuation of their earlier insights and directions, but quite clearly a distinct and important advance in our understanding of ethics: the incisive way in which major philosophical—but pre-eminently practical—insights are discovered within the wholly concrete life of nursing practice. Careful attention to their unfolding arguments makes very clear that no one profession could possibly have a lock on what ethics is all about.

Their practical, interpretive effort to disclose the ethical character of nursing requires careful attention be paid to its practice. By doing so, Bishop and Scudder continue and advance their fascinating and thoughtful voyage into one of the most concrete and distinctive regions of human life: the intimate, complex relationships among sick people and those who both care for them and seek to take care of them. It is a study that is most rewarding for its important insights into and understanding of ethics in its broader, if still deeply troubled, presence in our society.

—*Richard M. Zaner, Vanderbilt University Medical Center*

END NOTES

1. For instance, Ronald Munson, *Intervention and Reflection: Basic Issues in Medical Ethics*, Belmont, CA: Wadsworth, Inc. 4th edition, 1992, hardly has a word about nurses or their "ethics."
2. Alasdair MacIntyre, *After Virtue*, Notre Dame, IN: University of Notre Dame Press, 1982.
3. Albert R. Jonsen, Mark Siegler, William J. Winslade, *Clinical Ethics*, New York: McGraw-Hill, 1992.
4. Tom L. Beauchamp and James J. Childress, *Principles of Biomedical Ethics*, New York: Oxford University Press, 4th edition, 1994.
5. A notable exception is an anthology edited by Anne H. Bishop and John R. Scudder, Jr.: *Caring, Curing, Coping: Nurse, Physician, Patient, Relationships*, University, AL: University of Alabama Press, 1985.

6. Sally Gadow, "Existential Advocacy: Philosophical Foundation of Nursing," in S. Spicker and S. Gadow (eds.), *Nursing: Images and Ideals: Opening Dialogue with the Humanities*, New York: Springer, 1980.
7. Patricia Benner, *From Novice to Expert: Excellence and Power in Clinical Nursing Practice*, Menlo Park, CA: Addison-Wesley, 1984.
8. Anne H. Bishop and John R. Scudder, Jr., *The Practical, Moral, and Personal Sense of Nursing: A Phenomenological Philosophy of Practice*, Cf. p. 227 Albany, NY: State University of New York Press, 1990.
9. Anne H. Bishop and John R. Scudder, Jr., *Nursing: The Practice of Caring*, New York: The National League for Nursing Press, 1991.
10. Nel Noddings, *Caring: A Feminine Approach to Ethics and Moral Education*, Berkeley, CA: University of California Press, 1984.
11. Carol Gilligan, *In A Different Voice: Psychological Theory and Women's Development*, Cambridge, MA: Harvard University Press, 1982.
12. E. R. DuBose, R. Hamel and L. J. O'Connell (eds.), *A Matter of Principles? Ferment in U.S. Bioethics*, The Park Ridge Center for the Study of Health, Faith and Ethics, Valley Forge, PA: Trinity Press International, 1994.
13. Richard M. Zaner, *Ethics and the Clinical Encounter*, Englewood Cliffs, NJ: Prentice Hall, 1988.

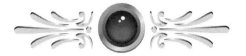

FOREWORD TO SECOND EDITION

The revised second edition of Anne Bishop and John Scudder's book, *Nursing Ethics*, is an insightful exploration of the moral practice of nursing. Beginning with the assertion that there is an inherent moral sense in nursing practice, they have revitalized the discussion of nursing ethics by placing it within the context of nursing practice—exactly where it belongs. How did nursing ethics stray from its rightful place for so long? One reason is nursing's apparent fascination with medical ethics and the application of traditional ethics to the realm of practice. While such an approach has an important role in applied ethics, it does not capture the holistic nature of nursing practice.

In this second edition of their book, Bishop and Scudder remind us that the situation of practicing nurses is an important aspect of nursing ethics. Unfortunately, this important aspect has been overlooked by merely applying traditional ethics to nursing practice. Crucial to Bishop's and Scudder's view of nursing ethics is the notion that the practice of nursing is a practice of caring. By this, they mean that the morally good nurse is motivated to care and to regard the patient as a whole person. By his/her caring presence, the morally good nurse even enhances patient well-being by fostering cooperation between those involved in the patient's care. While the authors no longer regard this view of nursing ethics as therapeutic, they still recognize it as contributing to the well-being of patients. When the sentiment of care is combined with the practice of care, the nurse is a morally good nurse. Nursing knowledge and skill are thus integrated with the practice of caring and center on the well-being of the patient.

This new edition of the book requires one to reconsider what it means to be a nurse. Rather than someone who simply applies ethical thinking in nursing practice, the nurse is a moral being who is engaged in a moral practice. Nursing ethics grows out of such a practice. On behalf of nurses everywhere, I thank them for reminding us of the moral sense inherent in nursing practice.

Sara T. Fry, PhD, RN, FAAN
Henry R. Luce, Professor of Nursing Ethics
Boston College School of Nursing

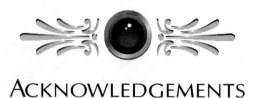

ACKNOWLEDGEMENTS

Portions of Chapter 3 were taken, with some revision, from
Bishop, Anne H. and Scudder, John R., Jr. (1997). A phenomenological interpretation of holistic nursing. *Journal of Holistic Nursing.* 15,(2), 103–111.

Bishop, Anne H. and Scudder, John R., Jr. (1999). A philosophical interpretation of nursing. *Scholarly Inquiry for Nursing Practice*, 13 (1), 17–27.

Portions of Chapter 4 are from
Noddings, Nel. *Caring: A Feminine Approach to ethics*, 1984. University of California Press. Copyright University of California Press. Used with permission of University of California Press.

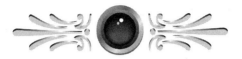

Table of Contents

1
Why Another Nursing Ethics Book?	1
Dialogical Interpretation	4
Study Hints for This Book	14
Study Questions	14
References	15

2
On Being a Good Nurse	17
Examples of Basic Nursing	17
Integral Nature of Nursing Practice	19
An Outstanding Nurse	21
Example of Trish as an Outstanding Nurse	21
The Moral Sense of Competency	23
Example of CPR	23
From Competency to Excellence	24
Practical Wisdom	25
Example of Nancy and Young Physician Patient	25
Good Nurses, Not "The Good Nurse"	26
Study Questions	27
References	28

3
Wholistic and Holistic Care	29
Margie Smith and Mrs. Cooper	29
Wholistic Care	33
The Moral Imperative to Reform Health Care	34
Holistic Care	35
Claire Hastings and Woman with Arthritis	35

Study Questions	39
References	39

4

Caring Presence	41
Buber: Personal Relations	43
Example of Sarah	43
I-It (Thou) Relationships	46
Triadic Dialogue	47
Noddings: Caring	48
Natural Caring in the Ethical	50
Conflicting Moral Desires and Limited Time	51
Caring in Practice	52
Zaner: Caring Response to Presence	55
Reflexive Presence to the Lived Body	55
Example of Sam	56
Vivid Presence	57
Nurse Extern Example	58
Barbara Ball and Mrs. Frazier	58
Co-Presence	60
Concluding Exemplar: Midori and Beverly	61
Study Questions	63
References	64

5

Called to Care	67
Being Called to Care: Peggy Chinn	67
The "Of Course" Response to Calls to Care	69
Pellegrino: The Call of Profession	70
James: Concrete Calling	71
Jesus: Called by the Plight of the Neighbor	72
Werner Marx: Called by Compassion	73
Example of Nurse with Dying Woman	75
Taylor: The Call to Authenticity	75
The Integral Calling of Compassion and Authenticity	81
Study Questions	82
References	83

6	THE ETHICAL IN HOLISTIC PRACTICE	85
	ZANER'S CLINICAL ETHICS	85
	ZANER'S REQUIREMENTS FOR CLINICAL ETHICS	86
	EXAMPLE OF TOM AND ZANER	87
	EXAMPLE OF LARA AND ROBIN	92
	EXAMPLE OF BARBARA AND HER PATIENT	95
	EXAMPLE OF MR. JONES AND MARY	96
	ETHICS IN HOLISTIC CARE	98
	STUDY QUESTIONS	100
	REFERENCES	101
7	REFLEXIVE DIALOGUE ON ETHICS AND NURSING	103
	REFLEXIVE DIALOGUE	105
	ON BEING A GOOD NURSE	106
	WHOLISTIC AND HOLISTIC CARE	107
	CARING PRESENCE: MIDORI AND BEVERLY	111
	CALLED TO CARE	112
	AN ETHICS OF PRACTICE	116
	CONCLUDING DIALOGUE	119
	STUDY QUESTIONS	120
	REFERENCES	121

APPENDIX   123

INDEX   133

CHAPTER

WHY ANOTHER NURSING ETHICS BOOK?

Nurses, physicians, and other medical professionals have recently turned to ethicists for help in resolving moral problems that have resulted from the complexity of modern health care. Most nursing ethics books focus on these moral problems and how philosophical ethics can help resolve them. In contrast, this book was initiated by new understanding of the meaning of nursing. This new understanding emerged from a reinterpretation of the meaning of nursing as a caring practice. This reinterpretation calls for a nursing ethics that takes seriously the meaning inherent in nursing practice. Nursing traditionally assumed that it was a caring practice, but that assumption was neither adequately probed nor articulated. The current reinterpretation of nursing is focused on recovering the initial meaning of nursing as a caring practice with an emphasis on the deeper meaning of the profession. We have taken part in this development by interpreting nursing first as a practice with an inherent moral sense (Bishop & Scudder, 1990) and then as the practice of caring that fulfills that moral sense (Bishop & Scudder, 1991). Then we developed an ethic that is rooted in the moral sense of nursing (Bishop & Scudder, 1996). This book is a revised second edition of that book that incorporates significant changes as indicated by the changing of the subtitle from "Therapeutic Caring Presence" to "Holistic Caring Practice."

We believe that nursing needs to develop its own ethics focused on nursing practice and the fulfillment of its moral sense, rather than merely applying philosophical ethics to moral problems. In taking this position, we are not denying the important contribution that applied ethics has made and is making to nurses who face moral problems. Instead, we are advocating a new approach to nursing ethics that speaks directly to the situation of practicing nurses by taking seriously the moral intent of nursing practice.

This book on ethics is a continuation of our previous work, which has attempted to examine nursing in a way that helps nurses become better nurses. We have contended that nursing is a practice with an inherent moral sense. Nursing is neither a theoretical activity nor a practical activity in the limited sense of "tricks of the trade." Nursing does not begin with theory that is applied to the world to achieve certain ends. Instead, it is a practice in that it is made up of practical ways of fostering the good—that is, the well-being—of persons. Although it is a practice, it is not practical in the limited sense that it has been for much of the twentieth century. Historically, nursing was taught primarily as techniques and procedures that had to be followed precisely, with little attention to the context of meaning. As nursing developed, an attempt was made to supply the context of meaning from nursing theories drawn from outside nursing. Although we have been critical of this approach to nursing in our books, these theories did move nursing beyond techniques and procedures. Unfortunately, these theories not only moved thought about nursing away from practice, but also moved it away from the moral sense in which that practice is rooted. And it is that moral sense that has to be at the root of any nursing ethics.

We will attempt to develop a nursing ethics that is rooted in the moral sense of practice. This approach is different from the typical biomedical approach, in which ethical issues are generally considered to result from advances in modern technology. The biomedical ethics approach implies that medicine, and perhaps nursing, is a technological activity that occasionally generates moral problems that require the help of experts called *ethicists*. These experts usually apply ethics to nursing problems by converting nursing problems into ethical issues as formulated by philosophers. Practical problems and dilemmas taken from practice are often used to illustrate how to employ philosophical norms and reasoning, rather than how to achieve the good at which the practice aims. Books on medical and nursing ethics are replete with such examples. Usually, they are carefully selected to illustrate the importance of applied ethics and the use of philosophical norms and reasoning to resolve moral problems in health care.

In the applied approach, the emphasis is usually on whether the action taken coheres with ethical principles, such as autonomy or utilitarianism, rather than on fostering the well-being of the patient. Thus, ethics is primarily concerned with taking action that conforms to an ethical principle, rather than fostering the well-being of patients. Nursing needs an approach to ethics that takes seriously the moral sense of nursing and thus speaks directly to practitioners.

It was this insight that initially led us to write our first book on nursing ethics, of which this is a revised second edition. The emphasis on the moral sense of nursing was so pronounced in one of our earlier books (Bishop & Scudder, 1990) that it was twice reviewed as a book on nursing ethics. However, that book was not about nursing ethics; rather, its intent was to argue that nursing was a practice with an inherent moral sense. Rather than developing an ethics of nursing, we merely asserted that any nursing ethics had to be rooted in that moral sense. In this book, we will continue to develop a nursing ethics that is rooted in the moral sense of nursing.

Neither of us is a specialist in ethics, applying his or her expertise to nursing. We are, instead, interpreters of nursing who have been led into nursing ethics by the moral sense we found inherent in nursing practice. This approach has the strength of being closely tied to nursing as practiced and of speaking directly to nurses engaged in practice. It has a weakness, however, in that we have not, over our careers, been preoccupied with health care ethics, and specifically with nursing ethics. Our colleague, Sara Fry, is such a specialist in nursing ethics. For that reason, she wrote the article concerning nursing ethics for the *Encyclopedia of Bioethics* (Fry, 1995), in which we wrote the other two articles on nursing, one on the philosophy of nursing (Bishop & Scudder, 1995) and the other on nursing as a profession (Bishop, 1995). In Fry's contribution to that encyclopedia, she gives an overview of nursing ethics that we have included as an appendix for the convenience of our readers. Here we consider two aspects of her treatment of nursing ethics that speak forcefully to our interpretation of nursing ethics.

First, she points out that the crucial conflict in contemporary nursing ethics concerns whether nursing ethics has "a distinct voice in health care" or is merely a "subcategory of medical ethics." Those who believe "there is little that is morally unique in nursing practice" regard nursing ethics as a minor aspect of medical ethics, which in turn is a part of applied ethics. Those who hold the former view believe that "the moral concepts and obligations inherent in nursing practice are different from (yet compatible with) those in other health care professions" (Fry, 1995, p. 1826) and, hence, a nursing ethic is needed.

Those who are attempting to develop a nursing ethic, according to Fry (1995), have focused on advocacy, accountability, collaboration, and caring. In this text, we treat advocacy in the context of being authentic; we contend that nurses are accountable for the moral responsibilities inherent in nursing practice; and we stress collaboration in our treatment of wholistic nursing. The thrust of our ethic, however, is caring and practice and the integral relationship between them. When we consider advocacy, accountability, and collaboration, we do so within the context of the practice of caring, which for us is the essential meaning of nursing.

Our ethics of the practice of caring is initiated in Chapter 2, in which we discuss the meaning of being a good nurse. In good nursing, the motivation to care and the practice of care are integrally related. In Chapter 3, a new chapter, we explore holistic care, in which nurses as whole persons care for patients as whole persons. In wholistic care, we consider how nurses enhance patient well-being by fostering cooperation among those involved in health care. In Chapter 4, we describe, illustrate, and articulate the caring presence that is an essential aspect of any caring ethics in nursing. Originally, we had intended to write our first ethics book on caring presence, but we discovered that caring presence, even when predicated on the moral sense of nursing practice, could not adequately encompass nursing ethics. A nursing ethics needs to treat the call to care and how that call is inherent in nursing practice. In Chapter 5, we interpret that call philosophically in a way that does not require religious calling but does not exclude it.

In Chapter 6 of our first edition, we attempted to show that any adequate nursing ethics is therapeutic. We came to this conclusion by recognizing how Richard Zaner's work as an ethicist often contributed directly to the well-being of patients. We now believe that it was a mistake to refer to his clinical ethics as a "therapeutic" ethic. We believe that it is more correct to speak of the positive contribution ethics makes to recognizing and fulfilling the moral sense of nursing practice. We attempt to show how ethics makes a positive contribution to the well-being of patients by interpreting several examples of practice. The concluding chapter, Chapter 7, begins with a brief summary of the book. Then it shifts to a dialogue between the authors. The purpose of that dialogue, as well as that of this book, is to explore the possibility of an ethics that grows out of the moral sense of nursing, one that helps practicing nurses recognize and realize the moral sense of practice. This dialogical approach allows the authors to speak from their individual perspectives, rather than from the common perspective usually expressed as "we." Anne, one of the authors, speaks from the perspective of a practicing nurse with extensive experience in nursing education and a clinical specialty in psychiatric nursing. Jack, the other author, brings to their dialogue the perspective of a philosopher who, as a specialist in phenomenology of the human sciences, has written extensively in the philosophy of education. Although both are committed to feminist values, they speak from long experience of situations in which the separation of men and women and male dominance were taken for granted. For over twenty years, they have engaged in an on-going dialogue concerning the meaning of nursing, in which each of the partners speaks out of his or her own particular experience. Because this dialogue is a personal one as well as one between a philosopher and a nurse, we have chosen to designate the participants personally as Jack and Anne. We will initiate this dialogical approach in the remainder of this chapter and then return to it in the final chapter.

DIALOGICAL INTERPRETATION

Jack: I think that the way you became involved in ethics is more interesting than my involvement in ethics. After all, ethics is one of the primary fields of interest of philosophers.

Anne: It is difficult to be a nurse and not consider moral issues. I know it is fashionable to say that interest in ethics came from advances in biomedical technology, but nursing, as I have known it, always involved moral concerns.

Jack: Advances in biomedical technology could not be the source of moral concerns in nursing if, as we claim, nursing has an inherent moral sense. However, advances in biomedical technology have certainly made health care workers more aware of the moral issues inherent in their practice.

Anne: When these issues became urgent, nurses turned to philosophers for help. I suppose that's why books on nursing ethics have tended to be applied ethics.

Jack: As I remember it, your first encounter with philosophical ethics took the applied approach.

Anne: Yes, I used one of the first texts that applied philosophical ethics to nursing ethics during a seminar designed to introduce nursing leaders to ethical thinking.

Jack: I remember when you returned from the seminar. You proudly asserted that now you were ready to argue with me about ethical issues in nursing.

Anne: Then you asked a crucial question: Did the work of the seminar prepare me to help nursing students recognize and resolve the issues they face in nursing practice? I responded, "No," but I think that you already knew that I would.

Jack: I remember all your frantic phone calls requesting help in understanding the meaning of Kantian autonomy and utilitarianism. It sounded like a typical course in ethics taught by a philosopher, and I remember wondering how it was specifically related to nursing practice. That's why I asked you whether it would help you introduce nursing students to ethical issues confronted in nursing practice.

Anne: In the seminar, we examined problems that were supposedly typical of the ethical problems that nurses face in practice. Autonomy ethics and utilitarian ethics sometimes seemed to speak to some of these problems.

Jack: With all the emphasis on patients' rights, I can see why an autonomy ethics would speak to certain kinds of problems. These problems often deal with situations in which what the patient wants conflicts with what the nurse or physician thinks is best for the patient's health. Advocates of patients' rights draw on Kant because Kant insisted that every human being should be treated as an end, never merely as a means, and that making moral decisions required freedom to make the decisions.

Anne: The patient rights movement assumes that all patients have the right to decide what will be done to them, even when it goes against the best health care practice.

Jack: Advocates of utilitarianism often find themselves in conflict with advocates of rights. The utilitarian believes that we should make decisions that foster the greatest good for the greatest number. Often this means denying the rights of a particular patient for the good of all.

Anne: Didn't you once refer me to an article in which an ethicist used autonomy ethics as well as utilitarian ethics to argue against allowing a patient to decide not to be treated?

Jack: That article came from a book that was specifically designed to demonstrate the contribution of applied philosophy to various types of human endeavors (Perry, 1989). In that example, Perry, a medical ethicist, is confronted with an unusual case. A patient who had been admitted to the hospital with a broken bone began to engage in bizarre behavior. An examination of his records showed a past history of mania that had been successfully treated with lithium. When the patient was given lithium, he became rationally competent to make decisions. In a rational state, he demanded that the lithium treatment be stopped, because he enjoyed being in the manic state. An ethicist was called in to assess the moral issues involved in this case. The ethicist considered the case from the point of view of both utilitarianism and Kantian autonomy. After arguing that utilitarianism would favor treatment, he then considered Kantian ethics. First, he argued that a Kantian autonomy ethics favored non-treatment because the patient, while in a rational state, decided he did not want to be treated. Then the ethicist raised the issue of whether a person has the right to use autonomy to deny any possible future autonomy. If autonomy or self-direction is the highest good, can one legitimately use this claim to preclude future ability to make autonomous decisions? Ethicists often treat this problem as the issue of "does one have the right to sell oneself into slavery?" The ethicist in this case concluded that one does not have such a right, and therefore the patient should be treated.

Anne: Did the physicians follow the ethicist's recommendation?

Jack: No, they ignored both arguments.

Anne: I'm not surprised, since he completely failed to address the clinical situation. What decision did the physicians make?

Jack: They decided to treat the patient on the basis of third-party considerations, namely, that non-treatment would impose an undue burden on the family and health care facilities. In presenting this case as an example of applied ethics, the ethicist did not even raise the issue of why the physicians ignored his ingenious and well-developed arguments.

Anne: Wasn't he concerned about how the physicians arrived at their decision or the adequacy of their decision?

Jack: No, he didn't discuss either. But it seems clear that the physicians as practitioners were primarily concerned with the well-being of the patient and those who must care for him, and not with ingenious philosophical arguments.

Anne: I think that the physicians were right in being concerned with the well-being of the patient and those who cared for him. Nursing needs an approach to ethics that speaks directly to practitioners and takes seriously the moral sense of nursing.

Jack: Does this mean that you think that the applied approach has little to offer nursing?

Anne: No. I think I benefited greatly from participating in a seminar on the applied approach. But I do not believe that the applied approach should be the only approach. Moral decisions are required by the nature of nursing practice, and nurses are continually faced with decisions of moral import. My concern is that those who use the applied approach tend to neglect the process of nursing. For example, nursing usually involves an ongoing process in which there is continual interaction between the patient and nurse, not with problems that can be solved in a once-and-for-all fashion.

Jack: It seems to me that what's often called a moral *problem* in nursing could more appropriately be called a moral *dilemma*. In nursing practice, aren't nurses more often confronted with moral situations and dilemmas than with moral problems?

Anne: Yes. Most issues in nursing ethics cannot be solved as problems, but must be responded to in ongoing situations. In these ongoing situations, there are possibilities for expanding and enhancing client well-being. In a problematic approach, nurses look for solutions rather than for possibilities that enhance and expand the practitioner's ability to foster patient well-being in an ongoing and developing process.

Jack: Most of the cases I've examined in nursing ethics books are chosen to illustrate types of philosophical thinking rather than issues encountered in typical nursing practice.

Anne: Many cases chosen for ethical examination refer to a past situation. Nurses are concerned with present decisions, actions, and interpersonal relationships that are directed toward improving future health, not with what has happened in the past. And even when these cases are directed toward the future, they are treated as if a once-and-for-all decision is going to be made. For example, there is much talk in health care ethics about informed consent. The pattern for informed consent seems to come from granting permission to perform medical or surgical procedures.

Jack: Do you mean that the patient signs a form that says to the physician, in effect, that it is okay to "do it to me?" Of course, such consent assumes that I have been informed about what will be done to me and the risks involved.

Anne: The "do-it-to-me" aspect of informed consent assumes that this is a once-and-for-all procedure, such as having your appendix removed. Informing consent makes more sense in nursing practice than informed consent. Nurses have to continually inform patients about what they are going to do to and with them, and continually need their tacit, if not explicit, consent. The purpose of informing consent is to foster cooperative relationships between patient and nurse, not merely to respect patient rights. Cooperative relationships are required for healing to take place, for pain to be relieved, or for hope to be restored.

Jack: Informing consent might also make more sense than informed consent in medical ethics. Regardless, the appropriateness of informing consent for nursing practice indicates why nursing ethics should take seriously the way in which nursing is practiced.

Anne: In fact, our concern with ethics has grown out of our attempt to make sense out of nursing as it is practiced. In our previous books, we have shown not only that nursing is a practice with an inherent moral sense, but that most nurses, at least implicitly, recognize that moral sense.

Jack: Most human endeavors have a dominant sense, which is only sometimes a moral one. In a free enterprise economy, the dominant sense of business is making profit for the owners. In business, ethics concerns matters that are adjunct to profit-making. For example, business ethics asks how much a business can pollute the environment or endanger workers and clients in pursuing profit.

Anne: If, in business, ethical issues are adjunct to profit-making, those in business with strong moral commitments are in a tenuous situation.

Jack: Let me illustrate with an example. I attempted to purchase a used car to replace the old car with which I "limped" through graduate school. I asked a friend, who was in charge of sales for a car dealer, to find me a used car that I could afford. My friend took me to the used car lot and told me that he would not sell me any car on the lot because I was his friend, but he would find me a good affordable car. As we left the lot, my friend posed his dilemma: "I have to sell all of those cars at a profit. The well-being of my family depends on it. You are supposed to know about ethics. Tell me how I can do that and live by the Golden Rule?" My friend's dilemma resulted from being committed to an ethics that required him to help others, while his occupation required him to make as much profit as possible for his employers. Unlike my friend, a nurse engages in a practice that is designed to foster the well-being of others. That's one meaning of nursing's having a dominant moral sense.

Anne: But that does not imply that nurses do not face moral tension in trying to fulfill the moral imperative. A nursing scholar once used this tension to challenge an assertion I made that nursing is a practice with a dominant moral sense. She stated, "Practicing nurses feel guilty when they view your philosophy of nursing as nursing's having a moral sense!" And then she asked, "What happens when nurses can't always practice morally?"

Jack: That is a strange response to our contention that nursing has a dominant moral sense.

Anne: Nurses feel guilty because they know that much of what they do has direct and indirect effects on patient well-being. When they fail to fulfill the moral obligation, they feel guilty. This guilt is often dulled by routine procedures and technical and professional language that obscure the moral sense. Nurses feel less guilty when they can say, "I did this according to standard procedures," or "I did it using the latest technology" rather than "I'm morally responsible for ensuring that my care fosters the well-being of my patient." The guilt that nurses feel, when they recognize the inadequacy of their care, results from being engaged in a practice that positively seeks to foster the well-being of others. Our emphasis on the moral sense makes nurses aware of their moral responsibility.

Jack: My friend, the used car salesman, would gladly face the guilt that nurses face. He would like nothing better than to be in a profession that calls for fostering the well-being of others, and hence matches his Christian morality. My friend would think it strange that nurses feel guilty when they discover the moral sense of nursing. Given his commitment to foster the well-being of others, my friend would find it fulfilling to be in a practice in which he could be an excellent practitioner and, at the same time, fulfill his moral commitment to the well-being of others.

Anne: An ethics for nursing should be different from a business ethics, but I believe that in some ways they are becoming similar.

Jack: Is that because of the emphasis on balancing the budget in hospitals and other health care institutions, and the fee system used in paying physicians and others?

Anne: Those are significant factors, but that's not primarily what I had in mind. Often I have the feeling that nurses and physicians talk and sometimes act as if they are engaged in a purely professional or technical activity, and that moral issues arise as secondary concerns in the same way that they do in business.

Jack: That certainly matches the tendency of some bioethicists to approach ethical issues as if they result primarily from advances in modern technology. This, of course, implies that medicine, and perhaps nursing, is a technological activity that occasionally spawns moral problems that require the help of ethicists.

Anne: When nursing is regarded as a technological activity, then moral concerns become adjunct to that activity, as they are in business. When the primary sense of an activity, such as nursing, is a moral sense, moral considerations are the primary concern and focus.

Jack: Because this is so, an ethics suitable to nursing should emphasize actual cases that disclose how the moral imperative of nursing is fulfilled. In attempting to disclose the moral sense of nursing, we have interpreted many different examples of good nursing in our previous articles and books. This book will expand that articulation of the moral sense of nursing by considering examples that show the ethical import of fulfilling the moral imperative.

Anne: I don't see how we could adequately treat nursing ethics without interpreting examples of good nursing that disclose how the moral sense of nursing is realized. Nurses make many moral decisions each day concerning practice. Examples from practice can disclose how the moral demands of practice can be fulfilled in ways that will encourage better practice.

Jack: Our stress on concrete examples should not imply that we neglect philosophical treatments of the meaning of human being. Philosophy can enhance our understanding of the meaning of nursing and nursing ethics. Disclosing meaning through examples is sound philosophy, if we follow Paul Ricoeur's brief definition of phenomenology. He contends that phenomenology is a philosophy primarily concerned with disclosing meaning, that meaning is given as essence, and that essence is disclosed through well-chosen examples. Martin Heidegger has contributed to understanding the meaning of nursing by describing humans as beings who must care for themselves by projecting themselves into the world. They are able to do this by appropriating ways-of-being left to them by preceding generations. Nursing practice can be interpreted as "ready-to-hand" ways-of-being in the world that make it possible to care for self and others. A practice, as interpreted by Hans George Gadamer, one of Heidegger's disciples, is especially well-suited to articulate the meaning of nursing. He contends that a practice is a way-of-being-in-the-world developed over time that has as its goal fostering human well-being. In a practice, the way-of-being and the well-being sought are integrally related to each other. The way-of-being of nursing is caring, and the end of nursing is care that fosters well-being. Our interpretation of nursing as a practice with an inherent moral sense drew heavily on Gadamer's philosophy.

Anne: Patricia Benner's interpretation of nursing helped tie that philosophy of practice directly into nursing. Also, our contention that nursing is the practice of caring drew on the feminist philosophies of caring of Carol Gilligan and Nel Noddings.

Jack: But we have not attempted to found nursing on these philosophies. Instead, they enlightened our understanding of the meaning of nursing as practiced. In this book, Ricoeur, Heidegger, Gadamer, Gilligan, Noddings, Benner, Martin Buber, Richard Zaner, William James, Werner Marx, and Charles Taylor will enhance our understanding of nursing ethics.

Anne: What we mean by philosophy's enlightening our understanding of nursing is evident in how Gilligan contributed to our understanding of nursing care.

Jack: Gilligan supplied a context for what, in our first ethics book, we called the "in-between stance" in which nurses work: in-between physician, patient, and hospital administrator. We now call that stance *wholistic care*. Gilligan shows why this stance does not imply subservience to males. She argues that male thought is hierarchical and assumes that each person will strive to be alone at the top in order to be autonomous. In contrast, feminine values foster co-operation, interaction, and mutual support. Consequently, human beings should seek to practice wholistically, where they can support each other and foster cooperative interactions that promote each other's well-being.

Anne: Hierarchical systems based upon one highest value tend to distort nursing practice. In nursing as practiced, there are many values, some of which become more important than others in given contexts. For instance, a patient in excruciating pain wants more than anything else for the pain to end. A good nurse will usually do all that is possible to diminish the pain. That doesn't make the nurse or the patient a hedonist who contends that experiencing pleasure and avoiding pain are the highest good.

Jack: The fact that autonomy is of little concern to the patient who is enduring excruciating pain does not mean that autonomy is not to be highly prized in other circumstances.

Anne: Nurses value autonomy when physicians and hospital bureaucrats attempt to direct their nursing care. Nurses do need greater professional autonomy in order to bring about needed reform in patient care. Those seeking to reform nursing are understandably suspicious of a philosophy of nursing that reaffirms traditional nursing values. I can understand why our emphasis on deriving the meaning of nursing from actual practice has led many nurses to label us as "traditionalists." Nurses have struggled hard and long against a tradition that confined them—as nurses and as women—to a subservient role. They tend to hear valuing tradition as "traditional," even when the return to the past is a source of reform.

Jack: Most of the major reform movements, at least in the Western world, have come from seeing new possibilities in traditional values that have been neglected or distorted by changing times.

Anne: We nurses are recovering the centrality of caring in the nursing tradition that has been lost due to the emphasis on science, technology, and bureaucracy.

Jack: The emphasis on instrumental reasoning in technology and bureaucracy can obscure the moral sense, but caring discloses it.

Anne: The recovery of nursing as essentially caring is directing us to the moral sense of nursing as it is encountered in practice and shared with colleagues.

Jack: To hear some health care ethicists, you would think that advances in technology and bureaucracy created the need for ethics.

Anne: But they have the cart before the horse. Health care grew out of the need to care for the ill and debilitated in a given time and situation. In our time and situation, technological progress and administrative efficiency have become necessary for adequate health care. Although they have contributed much to the fulfillment of the moral sense of health care, they have, at the same time, tended to obscure the importance of the moral sense.

Jack: When people talk about advances in health care, they almost always speak of scientific and technological improvement. Why are the contributions of humanistic understanding of persons so often neglected?

Anne: It seems to me that nursing has been much improved by the emphasis on open disclosure, developing personal relationships, cooperative interactions, and authenticity.

Jack: Patients and their families have certainly benefited from such understanding. I remember when visiting a hospital was somewhat like entering an army post. You needed a pass to get in and children could not enter. Now hospitals are much more open.

Anne: Gaining information about treatment was almost impossible except when given by a physician in brief conferences full of technical language. Nurses never told patients what medications they were being given or what their blood pressure was. The only response the nurse could give was, "You'll have to talk to your doctor." Now, with the increased openness, nurses are able to discuss the meaning of illness and treatment with patients as human beings do in normal conversation.

Jack: Humanistic understanding has led to the recovery of the moral sense of nursing. Keeping the moral sense of health care focal is one of the most important contributions that ethics can make to health care.

Anne: I want that contribution to be focused on nursing as well as on ethics. When ethics concerns nursing, I want moral decisions, actions, and relationships to be considered as I encounter them in clinical situations.

Jack: When I do ethics, I want to consider something that's going on in the world that should foster the well-being of persons. When I teach ethics, I like to be philosophically engaged in exploring the meaning of the good as it is encountered in the world rather than as it has been distilled from the works of the great philosophers. My favorite ethics class was one in which our professor developed his own ethics and required us to explore and criticize the great classical ethical philosophies on our own. My only regret was that he did not give his ethics in written form so that it could be digested before class sessions, and its adequacy and possibilities be discussed in an ongoing dialogue in class.

Anne: When our book is used as a text, should it be used in the way you wish your professor had chosen? What difference does it make that those who use our book will not be its authors?

Jack: The issue, for me, is not who authored the text. I have used texts written by ethics professors that re-examined what past ethicists have said, criticized their ethics, and made suggestions for practical applications. Rather than taking that approach, my favorite professor invited us to think with him about the meaning of being moral in the world.

Anne: Our book is primarily an original interpretation of nursing ethics that begins with the moral sense of nursing. It is primarily directed toward the world rather than the classroom. Isn't it difficult for such a book to be a textbook? Didn't you and Al Mickunas run into a problem in trying to write a book that was a philosophical interpretation of education and at the same time a text?

Jack: We certainly did. Our editor demanded that we decide whether the book was a text or a contribution to knowledge. Because the book was about eighty percent contribution to knowledge and twenty percent text, it was not difficult for us to make the choice and eliminate the text-like chapter from the book. Seriously, that book, like this one, was not originally written as a textbook or a contribution to knowledge, although those who think in these terms would probably call it a contribution to knowledge.

Anne: I never thought of contributing to knowledge when we proposed this book. We wrote the book to explore the possibility of an ethics that grows out of and focuses on the moral sense of nursing. Such original explorations are usually aimed at specialists in colleges and universities, and are written in their customary language. We are attempting to avoid technical language and academic "insider" knowledge in order to speak to practicing nurses and students as well as scholars. Consequently, one answer to the question posed by the title of this chapter, "Why Another Nursing Ethics Book?" is that this book is different from books about ethics in that it is an original investigation of nursing ethics that seeks to involve students and nurses in that exploration.

Jack: I hope that, through sharing in our explorations, practicing nurses and students will recognize and realize the moral sense of their practice in ways that will enhance their abilities to engage in ethical considerations. By ethical considerations, I mean the ability to lift out the moral significance of their practice and to develop facility in understanding how to fulfill the moral imperatives in their practice. I also hope that students of ethics will learn to take seriously the moral sense embedded in practices.

Anne: I applaud the emphasis on understanding the ethical dimensions of practice, but I want more than understanding of the moral sense and its implications for practice. I hope that our articulation of nursing ethics will call nurses to thoughtful care for patients and for the practice of nursing. I especially want nurses to preserve the moral sense of practice that seems to be waning in this time of emphasis on technology and professionalism.

STUDY HINTS FOR THIS BOOK

Read the following chapters and answer the study questions at the end of each. After answering the questions, read the portion of Chapter 7 in which Anne and Jack engage in a dialogue concerning the major case or cases presented in the chapter in order to consider them in a broader ethical context. As you read the dialogue, questions or comments will come to your mind. Record these for consideration during class discussion. In the study questions we have also referred our readers to cases from Fry, S. T. and Veatch, R. M. (2000). *Case Studies in Nursing Ethics 2nd edition.* (Boston, MA: Jones & Bartlett) to give our readers an approach to ethics different from ours.

STUDY QUESTIONS

1. What are the major themes that Anne and Jack will develop in this book?
2. Why does Anne think that a traditional ethics focused on past cases is inadequate for making ethical judgments concerning nursing practice?
3. Why does Anne believe that informing consent is more appropriate for nursing practice than informed consent?
4. Why do some nurses feel guilty when reminded that nursing has a moral sense? Do you agree with them? Why or why not?
5. Why would the used car salesman who is committed to the Golden Rule find it strange that nurses feel guilty because nursing has a moral imperative?
6. Why does Anne believe that ethics in nursing is sometimes treated as it is in business?
7. What inadequacies in applied ethics are evident in the case of the ethicist who develops an ingenious argument from the principle of autonomy for treatment for the patient with mania?
8. Why do Jack and Anne believe that most moral problems in nursing ethics are more appropriately called moral *dilemmas*? For examples of dilemmas nurses face, see Case #4 and Case #53 in Fry & Veatch.
9. What do Anne and Jack mean by *practice*? Do you believe that nursing is a practice? Why or why not?

10. What reasons do Anne and Jack give for writing this book? What are some other reasons for writing a book on nursing ethics?
11. Why does Anne believe that nurses who stress autonomy tend to distrust reform based on return to traditional values?
12. Why do Anne and Jack favor the use of examples to disclose the meaning of being a good nurse?
13. Has the recovery of caring in nursing led to a recovery of the moral sense of nursing?
14. Why do Jack and Anne contend that humanistic understanding has led to the improvement of nursing care? Do you agree with their contention? Why or why not?
15. Why do Jack and Anne believe this book differs from traditional nursing ethics textbooks?
16. What do Anne and Jack hope will result from study of their book?

REFERENCES

Bishop, Anne H. (1995). Nursing as a profession. In Warren T. Reich (Ed.), *Encyclopedia of Bioethics*, (pp. 1827–1831). New York: Simon & Schuster Macmillan.

Bishop, Anne H., & Scudder, John R., Jr. (1990). *The practical, moral, and personal sense of nursing: A phenomenological philosophy of practice*. Albany, NY: State University of New York Press.

Bishop, Anne H., & Scudder, John R., Jr. (1991). *Nursing: The practice of caring*. New York: National League for Nursing Press, Jones and Bartlett.

Bishop, Anne H., & Scudder, John R., Jr. (1995). Nursing, Theories and Philosophy of. In Warren T. Reich (Ed.), *Encyclopedia of Bioethics*, (pp. 1818–1822). New York: Simon & Schuster Macmillan.

Bishop, Anne H., & Scudder, John R., Jr. (1996). *Nursing ethics: Therapeutic caring presence*. Sudbury, MA: Jones and Bartlett.

Fry, Sara T. (1995). "Nursing Ethics." In Warren T. Reich (Ed.), *Encyclopedia of Bioethics*, (pp. 1822–1826). New York: Simon & Schuster Macmillan.

Fry, S. T. and Veatch, R. M. (2000). *Case studies in nursing ethics* (2nd ed.). Boston, MA: Jones & Bartlett.

Gadamer, Hans-Georg. (1981). *Reason in the age of science*. (F. G. Lawrence, Trans.). Cambridge, MA: MIT Press.

Gilligan, Carol. (1982). *In a different voice: Psychological theory and women's development*. Cambridge, MA: Harvard University Press.

Heidegger, Martin. (1962). *Being and time*. (J. Macquarrie & E. Robinson, Trans.). New York: Harper and Row.

Noddings, Nel. (1984). *Caring: A feminine approach to ethics and moral education*. Berkeley, CA: University of California Press.

Perry, Clifton B. (1989). The Philosopher as Medical Ethicist: Applying Ethical Theories. In E. D. Cohen (Ed.), *Philosophers at work: An introduction to the issues and practical uses of philosophy*, (pp. 35–42). New York: Holt, Rinehart and Winston.

Ricoeur, Paul. (1977). Phenomenology and the social sciences. In M. Korenbaum (Ed.), *The annals of phenomenological sociology* II, (pp. 145–149). Dayton, OH: Wright State University.

Scudder, John R. Jr., & Mickunas, Algis. (1985). *Meaning, dialogue, and enculturation: Phenomenological philosophy of education.* Washington, DC: Center for Advanced Research in Phenomenology and University Press of America.

Zaner, Richard M. (1988). *Ethics and the clinical encounter.* Englewood Cliffs, NJ: Prentice Hall.

Zaner, Richard M. (1993). *Troubled voices: Stories of ethics and illness.* Cleveland, OH: Pilgrim Press.

CHAPTER 2

ON BEING A GOOD NURSE

It was after breakfast. I did not eat as much as I wanted to. I felt surprised, because I couldn't mobilize my will. I leaned back, as if I had used my body for hours. Suddenly she was there again, a nurse that had spent a lot of time with me the day before. She was smiling, full of energy. She went straight to the point, leaned on to the table and offered to help me have a shower in the bathroom. It seemed like climbing a mountain, but she was so convincing that I agreed. She explained the whole procedure, how she would cover the wound with plastic etc. It began sounding like heaven. I had confidence in her, she seemed to have been doing this for a hundred years. And it was heaven. Never had I thought that I would appreciate water running slowly down my body as I did that morning. I was sitting on a chair, and the nurse was next to me. I relaxed. She had a special way of offering her help in concrete ways like washing my back and my feet, which I literally could not reach that morning. "I suggest that you . . .," and "what you could do is turning your body . . .," yes she was assisting me, never taking over. I was in command, I felt. I mattered. Even though the only thing I could manage was steering the shower handle.*

The nurse in the preceding story (whom we will call Nancy) discloses the meaning of being a good nurse. Her care is good in both of the senses usually meant when nurses speak of "good nursing." Nancy is a good nurse in that her care is efficient, effective, and attentive, and because she acts out of the

---

*From *The world of the hospital nurse: Nurse patient interactions—body nursing and health promotion. Illustrated by use of combined phenomenological/grounded theory approach* by Ingegerd Harder. Copyright 1993. Aarhus, Danmarks Sygeplejerskehøjskole ved Aarhus Universitet, Skrift-serie fra Danmarks Sygeplejerskehøjskole 3/93, p. 173. Used with permission of Ingegerd Harder, R.N., Ph.D.

sentiment of care for this person in her situation. We contend that good nursing requires an integral relationship between the practice of care and the sentiment of care. Unfortunately, in contemporary nursing, these two senses are often separated. This separation of the practice of care from the sentiment of care often leads nurses to think of the ethical as concerning personal relationships and the practical as concerning technical methodology. We chose the above example because the knowledge and skill evident in it are those of basic nursing care. In the above case, knowledge and skill are so integrated with personal care that they may be unnoticed on first reading. Yet the confluence of knowledge and skill was recognized immediately by the patient as an integral ingredient in the liberating, comforting, and empowering care of her nurse.

Ingegerd Harder was struck by how well patients recognize the need for integral care in her study of patient response to basic nursing care. She found that although patients appreciated the sentiment of care, they were wary of nursing care that was strong on sentiment but weak on practice.

> That nurse had such a pleasant personality, she looked so kind, she was calm, she wanted me to feel comfortable, she wanted me to feel informed about what was happening. She was sort of 'serving' me, and she quietly organized my present world. But what about her failures, the times when she confused me, what about my feeling that she was not the most knowledgeable nurse? She left me in confusion a couple of times. But I liked her, she had a soothing effect on me. Her spontaneous warmth and calmness, I appreciated it so much.*

Patients recognized and appreciated competent, knowledgeable, efficient care even when the nurse was unable to establish a warm personal relationship.

> She had this efficient look about her. I did not feel rapport with her. Yet, I also knew that should things go wrong with me in some way or other, I would not mind her being on duty. She knew, she could cope in complicated situations. She made me unafraid.**

Although the nurse in the above example did not develop rapport with her patient, the patient did recognize the nurse's sentiment of care. She was unafraid because she knew that the nurse would use her skill and knowledge to care for her. That is one meaning of the *sentiment of care*. The other meaning is *personal care*, as evidenced in the following example.

---

*From *The world of the hospital nurse: Nurse patient interactions—body nursing and health promotion. Illustrated by use of combined phenomenological/grounded theory approach* by Ingegerd Harder. Copyright 1993. Aarhus, Danmarks Sygeplejerskehøjskole ved Aarhus Universitet, Skrift-serie fra Danmarks Sygeplejerskehøjskole 3/93, p. 172. Used with permission of Ingegerd Harder, R.N., Ph.D.

**From *The world of the hospital nurse: Nurse patient interactions—body nursing and health promotion. Illustrated by use of combined phenomenological/grounded theory approach* by Ingegerd Harder. Copyright 1993. Aarhus, Danmarks Sygeplejerskehøjskole ved Aarhus Universitet, Skrift-serie fra Danmarks Sygeplejerskehøjskole 3/93, p. 172. Used with permission of Ingegerd Harder, R.N., Ph.D.

She took care of me, she literally came very close to my body. I learned how much it means that someone really cares for my here-and-now comfort, for my physical well-being, which—I learned that, too—had a million positive effects on my more general well-being. She helped me with comfort and well-being.*

Patients are capable of distinguishing between *personable* care and *personal* care, and between being *likably* present and being *skillfully and knowledgeably* present. They associate good nursing with both personal and skillful-knowledgeable care, as Harder's study indicates. Patients experience good nursing as actual or potential attending to them. As Harder observed, good nursing often seems to the patient to have a "magical" quality: "I had a feeling that she was attending to me, even when she was not in the room for a while" (Harder, p. 173). This good nursing integrates the knowledge, efficiency, and effectiveness of the practice of care with the sentiments of care for the well-being of the patient and the patient as a person.

INTEGRAL NATURE OF NURSING PRACTICE

A crucial moral issue in nursing ethics concerns the relationship of *good* in the sense of attentive, efficient, and effective with *good* in the personal sense. Good in the first sense usually means understanding the ways of the practice of nursing and employing them to foster the well-being of patients. Good in the second sense usually means that nursing care grows out of personal concern for the well-being of patients. *Good* in the first sense becomes synonymous with *good* in the second sense when nursing is interpreted as a caring practice. A practice consists of historically developed ways of fostering good in which the good sought, the ways of fostering that good, and the personal concern for the other are integrally related to each other. Thus, to say that a nurse is morally good means he/she is actively concerned with fostering the patient's well-being through a caring relationship that requires attentive, efficient, and effective nursing practice.

Unfortunately, the personal aspect of nursing is often separated from the practical aspect and is regarded as the true meaning of the moral sense. This bifurcation was assumed by the nursing scholar mentioned in Chapter 1, who stated that nurses often feel guilty when morality is associated with sentiments, and they do not feel compassion for patients in their care. This separation of personal sentiments from the impersonal—the technological and

---

*From *The world of the hospital nurse: Nurse patient interactions—body nursing and health promotion. Illustrated by use of combined phenomenological/grounded theory approach* by Ingegerd Harder. Copyright 1993. Aarhus, Danmarks Sygeplejerskehøjskole ved Aarhus Universitet, Skrift-serie fra Danmarks Sygeplejerskehøjskole 3/93, p. 172. Used with permission of Ingegerd Harder, R.N., Ph.D.

professional—is unsound and detrimental to nursing practice. It reduces morality to personal relationships divorced from the empowerment of nursing practice. A morally good nurse would certainly cultivate the methods and skills necessary to empower effective care. In excellent practice, good nurses do not separate empowerment from personal sentiments. They show their personal concern for patients by supporting and empowering them so that they can recover from illness, overcome debilitation, and live more healthfully. When they engage in excellent practice, they are caring for the well-being of persons. Conversely, they care for persons by engaging in excellent practice.

When care for persons is separated from practice, a nurse is apt to say something like, "I care for the patient (I have a beneficent feeling toward the patient and therefore am a good, moral being) and therefore I must develop a nursing care plan" (I will be effective and efficient and therefore a good nurse). Nursing care does not happen in this way. When a nurse sees the patient in pain, she/he does not say, "I have a feeling of concern for this patient's well-being, therefore I must give the pain medication." She/he responds immediately to the pain with the prescribed remedy. If asked why the patient is being treated that way, the nurse would merely explain that the patient is in pain, rather than saying, "I have a beneficent feeling for the patient." The good of the patient is built into the remedy, and the nurse knows that it is. The ways of the practice have the good of the patient built into them; hence, they have an inherent moral sense. When they are employed, care for the person is present from the beginning. Of course, nurses are not always overtly conscious of this presence, but it is tacitly present in their actions.

In authentic nursing, good intentions are not separated from empowerment. When a nurse initially states, "I must do something to help this person," the empowering ability to do something is already present in her/his statement of commitment, although she/he may not be overtly conscious of it at the moment. What that empowering ability consists of depends upon the nurse and the situation.

When concern for well-being is separated from empowerment, then the moral good is usually limited to personal relationships from which empowering technical and professional competence are excluded. According to this way of thinking, the nurse is being moral when she/he cares for the patient personally, but not when she/he is efficiently using technology to foster the well-being of the patient. Nurses perform all kinds of activities efficiently and effectively that are not overtly connected to personal relationships or beneficent feelings. Nurses could hardly do otherwise. However, the well-being of the other is tacitly present in the activities and relationships that constitute nursing practice. Activities and relationships are moral in nursing when they are being done for the well-being of the other.

Many nurses see a clear relationship between morality and practice when personally attending to patients with the direct hands-on care that previously constituted much of nursing. But when engaged in complicated technological care, they find it difficult to recognize or feel the moral sense in that care. This is especially true in technical activities that require giving more attention to technique than to the patient. But nurses who work within the moral sense of practice recognize that temporarily focusing their attention away from the patient in order to perform exacting procedures is done for the good of the patient. It is not the nature of the activity—direct care or technical care—that makes it moral, but its being done for the well-being of the patient.

Because the moral sense is inherent in practice, it is possible for a nurse to contribute to fulfilling the moral sense of nursing without being a moral person. For example, consider a nurse who has concentrated on the practical aspects of nursing with limited understanding of the meaning of her/his work. Suppose also that the nurse works in a situation in which almost all of her/his work is prescribed by others, and that the nurse is primarily motivated by a desire to please superiors so that she/he can maintain employment and possibly be promoted. In this case, the nurse would have no intentional involvement in fulfilling the moral sense of nursing. This would mean that, although the nursing engaged in would have a moral sense, the nurse would not be a moral being when engaged in this moral practice. Such a nurse probably would consider herself/himself a moral being only when engaging in personal relationships with the right sentiments outside of her/his routine practice.

An Outstanding Nurse

The relationship of being a good nurse in the moral sense to that of being a good nurse in the practical sense has been disclosed in the writing and exemplars of Patricia Benner, to whom we are greatly indebted for contributions to the major thesis of this chapter and to our writings on nursing. We have chosen one of Benner's examples of nursing excellence to illustrate the integral relationship between being a good nurse in the practical and moral senses. She uses this example to illustrate excellent nursing in the domain of Effective Management of Rapidly Changing Situations. [The other domains are The Helping Role, The Teaching-Coaching Function, The Diagnostic and Patient-Monitoring Function, Administering and Monitoring Therapeutic Interventions and Regimens, Monitoring and Ensuring the Quality of Health Care Practice, Organizational and Work-Role Competencies (Benner, 1984, p. 46)].

> I came on duty at 3 PM and was assigned to a fresh postop open heart surgery. The patient had returned to the ICU around 11 AM that day and had all the usual paraphernalia for postops—IVs, respirator, chest tubes, foley catheters, etc. The patient had had a log [sic] of IV fluid and blood replacement on days—this is the usual procedure for open heart surgery—give lots of fluid at first (usually have had mannitol), then level off. Blood pressure will drop as the patient begins to warm up and dilate peripherally, but will usually level off soon. However, this patient continued to be hypovolemic—low blood pressure, low central venous

pressure—and was diuresing in enormous amounts. We were pouring fluids in, in an attempt to catch up, but were managing, barely, to stay even with output. The patient by this time (4:30-5 PM) was fully warm, so clearly something else was amiss here. I telephoned the surgeon's exchange but was not able to locate him. The exchange promised that they would have him call as soon as possible. I tried also to contact the assistant, but he was off call to another doctor who was not terribly familiar with open heart surgery. Meanwhile, we were pouring in fluids, blood and packed cells, without orders, just to stay even, for the patient was continuing this diuresis. I began reviewing the possible causes for this and decided a likely one was hyperglycemia. I then ordered a blood glucose level and the results came back—more than 600 mg percent. About this time the assistant surgeon had come back on call and I was finally able to contact him. He prescribed for the patient on the basis of the blood glucose level and we were then able to stabilize the patient.*

This is certainly an example of effective nursing, but it is also an example of morally good nursing. The nurse (whom we will call Trish) makes decisions and acts to foster the well-being of the patient. She gives the direction, without orders, necessary to keep her patient alive. When she is unable to secure a physician, she makes her own diagnosis and acts by ordering a blood glucose level.

But why does this make her a morally good person? She has not used the Kantian or utilitarian norms to make her judgment; in fact, these norms seem irrelevant to the many decisions she makes in response to changing conditions. She is a morally good person because she effectively decides and acts to foster the well-being of the patient. The goodness of her acts stand out, and therefore is outstanding, because she takes risks by proceeding without orders when they are unavailable but needed to foster the well-being of the patient.

Are only such outstanding decisions and acts moral care? Certainly not! By diligent and effective care, nurses continually foster the well-being of patients. Most nursing consists of just such care. But outstanding care makes the moral sense that is inherent in ordinary care stand out. Nurses are daily called on to routinely foster the well-being of patients. Only occasionally is that commitment tested by an unusual situation.

Trish could have failed the test by playing it safe. She could have reasoned that nurses should not act without medical orders, much less make diagnoses and issue orders. She probably would contend that a morally good nurse gives extra personal attention to patients. Consequently, she would hold the patient's hand, mop his brow, and pray for his well-being. However, her playing it safe would reveal that her primary concern is not for the well-being of the patient, but for legalistically "doing what nurses are supposed to do." Her decisions and actions would disclose her understanding of being a "good" nurse. For her, a good nurse stays safely within limits set by others and gives extra personal attention to the patient.

---

*From *From Novice to Expert* (pp. 116–117) by Patricia Benner, 1984, Menlo Park, CA: Addison-Wesley Publishing Company. Reprinted by permission.

But Trish did not do that. She took risks to foster the well-being of her patient. It is not taking risks that makes a nurse morally good, but rather the devotion to fostering the well-being of the patient that requires taking risks when the situation so demands.

THE MORAL SENSE OF COMPETENCY

Fulfillment of the moral sense of nursing occurs in competent care as well as in outstanding care. Much of the fostering of the well-being of patients by nurses occurs in competent care. When the implicit presence of "for the well-being of others" is obscured by work becoming routine or by a context of professional and technical non-moral systems of meaning, work becomes boring and burnout often occurs. An example of this is evident in the following description of a nurse's most fulfilling experience.

> The most fulfilling experience I ever had was when a child I was caring for arrested but was successfully resuscitated. I had written my notice that day—I wanted out of nursing—it was killing me. The baby stopped breathing while we were on the elevator coming back from X-ray. I did mouth-to-mouth on her until we got back to the room and the code team arrived. The baby responded beautifully. Naturally I felt good. But when the mother praised me for "saving" her baby, I tried to tell her that what I did was not so special; anyone can do mouth-to-mouth. "But it was you," she said. "You were there. If you hadn't wanted to be a nurse in the first place and been working that day, I wouldn't have my baby."*

The nurse in the preceding example decided to return to nursing when she recognized the moral sense inherent in competent nursing practice. Those who think that burnout comes from caring will find the above example strange. But it "is a peculiarly modern mistake to think that caring is the cause of burnout," according to Benner and Wrubel. They contend that, as the foregoing story discloses, "the return of caring is the recovery" from burnout (Benner and Wrubel, 1989, p. 373).

It is significant that, in the above example, the nurse's recovery from burnout occurred when she recognized the moral sense in competent care rather than excellent care. As the nurse said, "Anyone [presumably meaning any competent nurse] can do mouth to mouth." The mother's gratitude for the saving of her child led the nurse to recognize the moral sense inherent even in routine nursing practice. When this happened, the nurse recognized that the good in competent practice and the moral good were one and the same, and she decided to remain in nursing.

---

*From *The Practical, Moral, and Personal Sense of Nursing* (p. 101) Anne H. Bishop and John R. Scudder, Jr., 1990, New York: State University of New York. Reprinted by permission of SUNY Press.

From Competency to Excellence

The first moral obligation of a nurse is to become a competent practitioner. *Competency* refers to the minimum requirements for being a nurse. The primary obligation of nursing students and novice practitioners is to reach the level of competency. When nurses reach the level of competency, many are tempted to remain there rather than face the risks of authentic care. As Benner and Wrubel point out, "the risk and vulnerability inherent in caring lead to the temptation to create safe places of 'controlled caring' " (Benner and Wrubel 1989, p. 2). One of the safest places for a veteran nurse to control care is at the level of competent care. At that level care becomes routine and loses the connection with concern that was present when the nurse was striving for competency. Competent practicing nurses are morally obliged to become excellent practitioners. Being a good nurse implies moving beyond competency toward becoming an excellent practitioner.

Benner (1984) has interpreted becoming a good nurse as movement from novice to expert. She described this movement drawing on the work of Hubert Dreyfus and Stuart Dreyfus. Dreyfus and Dreyfus (1991) have shown that morality itself presupposes such a development. In evolving from novice to expert in ethics, persons first learn to follow the rules that commonly are regarded as the ethics of the community. Then, they act by following community maxims in the context of the situations in which they are involved. Finally, at the highest stage, rather than following the dictates of rules and principles, they make intuitive judgments concerning the right actions to take when encountering moral dilemmas and situations (Dreyfus & Dreyfus, 1991, pp. 236–237). Making intuitive judgments is recognizing the right thing to do without overtly going through all the rational processes involved in applying principles to practice.

Rather than following the traditional view that morally mature persons apply detached rational principles to moral problems, Dreyfus and Dreyfus contend that a morally mature person intuitively knows what to do, drawing from past experience. They also point out that a contextual intuitive ethics is the ethics of everyday moral life. This approach speaks directly to our attempt to develop an ethics that is appropriate to nurses in everyday practice.

This does not mean that learning to make moral judgments on the basis of principles is unimportant to the moral life. Novice nurses do need to learn how to make moral judgments, how to justify them rationally, and how to incorporate these abilities within their moral experience. Principled approaches to ethics teach nurses to value justice, rights, and autonomy, and to recognize situations in which justice, rights, and autonomy are involved, even when it is no longer necessary to follow them as principles that direct moral behavior. In clinical situations, nurses need to make intuitive decisions that draw on their past experience in order to foster the well-being of their clients. This moral experience needs to include the traditional moral wisdom of the community and ethical sensibilities developed during active participation in the moral life of that community.

The need to draw on general principles and common moral wisdom in making moral decisions should not keep nurses from consideration of the uniqueness of individuals and their situations, according to Dreyfus and Dreyfus.

> Each person must simply respond as well as he or she can to each unique situation with nothing but experience-based intuition as guide. Heidegger ... captures this ethical skill in his notion of *authentic care* as a response to the *unique*, as opposed to the *general*, situation. Authentic caring in this sense is common to *agape* and *phronesis*. (Dreyfus and Dreyfus, 1991, p. 246).

Caring that is activated by agape and informed by phronesis is well-suited for a nursing ethics. A*gape* is a selfless concern for the well-being of others and *phronesis* is practical wisdom that enables one to foster another's well-being.

Practical Wisdom

Because we are attempting to show that the know-how of nursing practice and that of nursing ethics are integrally related, we will focus on what philosophers have traditionally called "practical wisdom." A human activity is a practice, according to Gadamer (1981), when it is designed to foster human good. In that fostering of human good, the end sought and the way of achieving the good are one and the same. The Greeks used the word *phronesis* to refer to the know-how that fosters the good (Gadamer, 1981). Making both moral decisions and practical decisions in nursing require intuitive judgment that draws on experience. Benner (1984) has shown that making intuitive decisions by drawing on experience is characteristic of excellent nursing. This is evident in the following example of a nurse (whom we will call Betty) who let her physician-patient sleep rather than awakening him for chest physical therapy without certain knowledge that it would be more beneficial than physical therapy.

> I took care of a patient, a very likable young physician, who had an open-and-close exploratory laparotomy for pancreatic cancer. He had been febrile. For three nights I woke him every four hours and helped him do all his breathing exercises and lung physical therapy. He was really depressed and wasn't talking about anything that had to do with his diagnosis and everything that was happening to him. The fourth night that I was on, his temperature had come down some, and by now he was exhausted from lack of sleep. I figured that he was going to have a lot better chance to focus on things that he needed and wanted to focus on if he could just get some uninterrupted sleep. His temperature remained the same in the morning. His lungs probably would have been clearer had I awakened him at 3 AM but I elected not to, given his extreme fatigue and depression. It's not clear what is the right thing to do. There are little studies done about the effectiveness of

chest physical therapy and then there are other studies done about the effectiveness of sleep. But there is never anything that proves that X is better than Y, especially in a particular situation, so that I know that chest physical therapy every four hours is really going to help or that sleep is going to help. It is expected that I will use my best judgment under the circumstances.

In the preceding example, it is almost impossible to separate the moral from the practical. Betty is drawing on her past experience in making judgments concerning patient care that are at once practical and moral. This case is focused on how best to treat *this* particular patient in *this* concrete situation. In deciding what to do about this patient's sleep, Betty is not only concerned with his physical well-being, but also with his ability to make decisions about his future care. Just as there is no X or Y judgment demonstrating which decision is therapeutically best, there are no ways of making moral judgments that will clearly indicate which is the morally right course to follow in this case. Perhaps the best indication of Betty's high moral character is her willingness to make a judgment unsupported by rational props, when her long experience indicates that sleep is probably best for this particular person. Her outstanding care discloses the moral obligation for nurses to act intuitively and courageously to foster the well-being of the patient when thoughtful reflection indicates that it will, even though positive assurance is lacking.

Good Nurses, Not "The Good Nurse"

Nancy, Trish, and Betty are good nurses. Each is *a* good nurse, not *the* good nurse. We originally planned to discuss *the* good nurse in this chapter. But there is no *the* nurse. There are only Nancy, Trish, Betty and other nurses whose outstanding ways of being distinguish them as good nurses. Therefore, we have discussed the meaning of being *a* good nurse rather than *the* good nurse. I am a good nurse when my concern for patients is integrally related to efficient, effective, and attentive care that fosters their well-being. Even when I am not directly concerned about my patients' well-being, I am focused on ways of fostering their well-being because I am engaged in a practice with an inherent moral sense. The moral sense of nursing practice integrally relates concern with practical know-how. Nancy, Trish, and Betty reveal the meaning of being a good nurse by the way in which their effective, efficient, and attentive care is integrally related to their concern for the well-being of their patients.

From *From Novice to Expert* (pp. 140–141) by Patricia Benner, 1984, Menlo Park, CA: Addison-Wesley Publishing Company. Reprinted by permission.

Study Questions

1. What is the primary thesis of this chapter? How is this thesis illustrated in the bathing example that opens the chapter?
2. Why do Anne and Jack contend that nursing practice is distorted when the practical aspects of nursing are divorced from the personal? Do you agree? Why or why not?
3. Why is Trish's action in ordering a test for blood glucose level an example of outstanding nursing? Why is it also an example of outstanding moral action? What would Trish have disclosed as the meaning of nursing and morality by playing it safe? The example of the nurse we have called Trish is excerpted from Patricia Benner's *From Novice to Expert: Excellence and Power in Clinical Nursing Practice* (1984, pp. 116–117). Examine the exemplars in that book to find other examples of good nursing in which the practical and moral sense are integrally related and share them with your class. Also read "The Phenomenon of Caring," (pp. 170–173) in Benner's book for another context of good nursing as treated in this chapter.
4. Jack and Anne contend that burnout often occurs when nurses lose the moral sense of nursing. They provide the example of the nurse giving mouth-to-mouth resuscitation to support this contention. Does this example prove their contention, disclose the meaning of their contention, or prove that competent care is necessary? Why or why not?
5. Evaluate the movement from competence to excellence in ethics as described by Dreyfus and Dreyfus. Compare their beliefs to Benner's treatment of the movement from competence to excellence in nursing (Benner 1984). According to Anne and Jack, how are the two related?
6. Why do nurses need to act intuitively and courageously when faced with a perplexing moral decision? Do you believe that nurses have a moral obligation to act intuitively and courageously? If so, under what circumstances? For another case that raises this issue, see Fry & Veatch, Case #15.
7. What do Anne and Jack disclose in the example of Betty letting her patient sleep? Do you agree with their interpretation? Why or why not? Can you offer an alternative interpretation of the example?
8. Describe and interpret how the major themes of this chapter are illustrated in the cases of Nancy, Trish, and Betty. Could you also treat the same themes by discussing why they are good nurses?
9. Why did Anne and Jack call this chapter "On Being a Good Nurse" rather than "The Good Nurse?" Some philosophers argue that you could not know the meaning of being a good nurse without knowing what constitutes "the good nurse." Do you agree with Anne and Jack or the advocates of "the good nurse?" Why? Examine Chapter 7 for further consideration of why Jack and Anne stress the theme of being a good nurse in ethics.

REFERENCES

Benner, Patricia. (1984). *From novice to expert: Excellence and power in clinical nursing practice.* Menlo Park, CA: Addison-Wesley.

Benner, Patricia, & Wrubel, Judith. (1989). *The primacy of caring: Stress and coping in health and disease.* Menlo Park, CA: Addison-Wesley.

Bishop, Anne H., & Scudder, John R., Jr. (1990). *The practical, moral, and personal sense of nursing: A phenomenological philosophy of practice.* Albany, NY: State University of New York Press.

Dreyfus, Hubert L., & Dreyfus, Stuart E. (1991). Towards a phenomenology of ethical expertise. *Human Studies,* 14, pp. 229–250.

Fry, S. T., and Veatch, R. M. (2000). *Case studies in nursing ethics* (2nd ed.). Boston, MA: Jones & Bartlett.

Gadamer, Hans-Georg. (1981). *Reason in the age of science.* (F. G. Lawrence, Trans.) Cambridge, MA: MIT Press.

Harder, Ingegerd. (1993). *The world of the hospital nurse: Nurse patient interactions—body nursing and health promotion. Illustrated by use of a combined phenomenological/grounded theory approach.* Aarhus, Danmarks Sygeplejerskehøjskole ved Aarhus Universitet, Skrift-serie fra Danmarks Sygeplejerskehøjskole.

Chapter

Wholistic and Holistic Care

We will show why being a good nurse involves wholistic and holistic care by interpreting Margie Smith's (1993) wholistic and holistic care of Debra Cooper. Readers of our first edition of this book will recognize Margie as our example of a good nurse. The difficult circumstances of her outstanding care for Mrs. Cooper highlight the meaning of wholistic and holistic care and, at the same time, show the integral relationship between wholistic and holistic care.

Both holistic and wholistic care are concerned with treating the whole person. Wholistic care focuses on bringing together the diverse practices and sciences of health care into unified care. Holistic care focuses on bringing the sentiment of care and the practice of care together in a personal-professional relationship between nurse and patient that fosters the well-being of the patient as a whole person.

> Debra Cooper, 78 years old, was admitted to the geriatric rehabilitation unit with a left above-the-knee amputation which, like her right previous below-the-knee amputation (with a prosthesis), resulted from gangrene caused by Type I diabetes. She also had congestive heart failure and some disorientation as a result of organic dementia. Margie Smith was Mrs. Cooper's primary nurse.
>
> Before her left amputation, Mrs. Cooper was able to take care of herself and even help her daughter, who lived with her, with housekeeping, care of the 'grandbabies,' as she liked to refer to them, and cooking. Despite her disorientation, Mrs. Cooper knew she was in the hospital and that our job, in her words, was to "get me walking with my grandbabies again."
>
> After working with Mrs. Cooper for a few days I was impressed by her. She was one of the most motivated and cooperative patients I've ever known. Sure, she sometimes thought it was 1943, but she'd

learned how to get in and out of her wheelchair without having any legs, and could use the bedpan. She never stopped talking about her goal of walking with two artificial legs.

As I worked with her, I noticed that Mrs. Cooper's right prosthesis appeared loose. Her stump would twist within the prosthesis during transfers from the bed or wheelchair. It was loose enough that there were times when she would be standing almost literally on the ankle of her prosthesis as it tilted away from her stump. When I asked her about this, she admitted that the prosthesis "just didn't feel right."

When the occupational therapists confirmed Margie's observations regarding the prosthesis fit, she conferred with the physical therapist and physician, who disagreed and said nothing could be done. Margie was completely surprised when a discharge order was written for Mrs. Cooper after only one week and no team meeting to discuss her progress.

There hadn't been any attempt made to consult the prosthetist about Mrs. Cooper's ill-fitting right prosthesis or to fit her with a left prosthesis. There wasn't enough time to finalize the necessary discharge teaching with her daughter. More important, there was no wheelchair available for Mrs. Cooper and no time to teach this formerly ambulatory patient how to use it. Personally, I had difficulty turning this once-independent, ambulatory, motivated, cooperative woman, who was making good progress, into a wheelchair bound patient after only one week—especially on the basis of the physician's opinion alone. This wasn't the reason I went into nursing. This wasn't the standard of care I needed to give.

I talked about this with Mrs. Cooper's physician. His opinion was that Mrs. Cooper wasn't a good prosthesis candidate because of her disorientation. In response, I offered documented examples from all the nursing staff of Mrs. Cooper's ability to learn new skills and her extraordinary motivation to be independent. I also expressed concern over the fit of the right prosthesis and asked if the prosthetist had been consulted.

Despite his contention that Mrs. Cooper wasn't a good prosthesis candidate, he canceled the discharge order when Margie related that several members of the rehabilitation team had similar goals for Mrs. Cooper, including prosthetic and ambulation goals.

Margie and the occupational therapist continued to document major problems with the right prosthesis, while the physical therapist replaced Mrs. Cooper's stump socks with thicker ones every day or two. Although Margie requested a stump compression sock to begin preparing Mrs. Cooper for a left prosthesis, the physician or physical therapist did not agree that a left prosthesis was indicated in this case.

At the first team meeting, we found out that the physical therapist apparently had tried to have Mrs. Cooper "hop" between the parallel bars during the first few days of admission and she hadn't been able to hold herself up. I pointed out that Mrs. Cooper had lost some more fluid weight (10 pounds) in the last week and her congestive heart failure was more stable. Her endurance and strength had increased since then, too. I thought it was worthwhile to try the parallel bars again.

Within a few days Mrs. Cooper was hopping up and down the parallel bars, even though her right prosthesis remained awkward-looking. After this success, the physician finally agreed to order a consultation with the prosthetist. When the prosthetist attended the meeting, the team agreed that Mrs. Cooper was a prosthetic candidate.

I called the prosthetist a few days later to ask his opinion of Mrs. Cooper's right prosthesis because she was still having problems with it. Transfers were dangerous at times because she had to bear weight on an unstable prosthesis. The prosthetist said he hadn't been made aware of any right prosthesis problems, but that he'd assess the situation.

Three days later, as I was helping Mrs. Cooper off the toilet, her right leg came out of the prosthesis and I just managed to ease her to the floor. I immediately called the physical therapist, who told me she'd just changed the stump socks again that morning. This was obviously not enough. . . .

The next day the prosthetist adjusted the straps on Mrs. Cooper's right prosthesis. This worked for two or three days, but the 10-year-old straps stretched again and the problems continued. . . . Still, I was told repeatedly by other team members that "there's nothing that can be done" and "it's normal for this patient." I knew this wasn't true, but in their opinion I was "just the nurse, so I didn't know prosthetics." I continued to document my assessments as well as Mrs. Cooper's persistent complaints that the right prosthesis was "loose-fitting" and "not right."

Despite all this, Mrs. Cooper was walking 40 feet in therapy on both prostheses with a walker. Physical therapy and the physician's notes indicated "remarkable" and "amazing" progress. But it wasn't at all surprising to me.

During week five of Mrs. Cooper's stay, I did my biweekly duty of bringing up the right prosthesis fit problems with her physician. This time, however, I was told "It's being taken care of." The occupational therapists confirmed that they'd participated in a conversation with the prosthetist, physician, and the physical therapist about replacing the right prosthesis.

When I told Mrs. Cooper that she was going to get a new right prosthesis, she was quiet for a few moments. Then she turned to me and said, "Course you been sayin' that ever since we met." Within two days Mrs. Cooper had a brand new right prosthesis. Soon she was walking 300 feet with a walker.

I suppose this case study illustrates, once again, the problem of control and communication among health care professionals—and I'd prefer to spend my time relating positive team-building anecdotes.

But more importantly, this was a powerful reminder to all of us to listen to a patient's belief in herself.

Instead of focusing on Mrs. Cooper's deficits, the occupational therapists, the staff nurses, and I chose to focus on her many strengths. Her iron-willed determination and good humor were our greatest assets.

We were amply rewarded. I'm pleased that I was able to play an instrumental role in improving the quality of life for this patient.

What happened to Mrs. Cooper? After her two-week postdischarge appointment with her physician, Mrs. Cooper, using a walker, came to see me—with her beloved grandbabies in tow.*

This story portrays the nurse's wholistic role in fighting for care that fosters the patient's well-being, even against strong opposition and mistaken judgments from the patient's physician and physical therapist. It shows how a nurse can take a strong stance concerning patient treatment in opposition to other health care professionals and, at the same time, foster cooperative teamwork. It also demonstrates why once-and-for-all decisions are often inadequate and why a series of decisions and actions are required in light of changing understanding and circumstances. It shows how intuitive judgment that included such factors as a patient's strength and determination can be the basis for seeing new possibilities for patient well-being. In this case, Margie Smith is a morally good nurse because her concern for the well-being of the patient is embodied in efficient, effective, and attentive nursing that eventuates in successful therapy for Mrs. Cooper. Margie's concern is not for the abstract autonomous rights of the patient. Her care is holistic in that she cares for Mrs. Cooper as a person. She is so engrossed in Mrs. Cooper's situation that she knows what Mrs. Cooper wants and is capable of doing. Her personal relationship with the patient is not an add-on to her professional care, but is integrally related to her holistic care.

The purpose of the nurse's relationship with patients/clients is to foster their well-being, and this requires—as Margie Smith makes evident—placing professional care in the context of personal well-being. Such care is holistic in that it fosters the well-being of this patient in a way appropriate to this patient's unified experience of his/her own being. Holistic care involves the personal-professional relationship between patient and nurse. This holistic care requires wholistic care that brings together the relationship between nurses, patients, physicians, and other health care professionals, and is supported by family, community, and institutions. Wholistic care brings together that which has been separated and separates. We contended in the first edition of this book—and still believe—that nurses have a special responsibility to foster integral care among these entities, as well as contribute their nursing expertise to it. Unfortunately, we have in the past labeled this responsibility

---

*From "Two Legs to Stand On" by Margie Smith, 1993, *American Journal of Nursing*, 93, p. 22. Used with permission. All rights reserved.

the *in-between stance*. (Bishop & Scudder, 1990) We now recognize that this term has negative connotations that evoked unnecessary controversy in the nursing community. We now use the term *wholistic care* to designate nursing that unifies all patient care with the patient's desire and aspirations.

WHOLISTIC CARE

Nurses, more than other health care workers, are aware of the need for cooperative interaction and are better prepared to foster it because they are in a position to coordinate the patient's whole care. Wholistic care is day-to-day care through which nurses foster their patients well-being by bringing together nursing care, the physician's plan of medical care, the institution's policies and resources, and the patient's view of the good life (Bishop & Scudder, 1990).

Carol Gilligan (1982) gave us a context for wholistic care. She interpreted care as fostering a web of connection. Gilligan has contended that traditional ethics has had a masculine hierarchical order rather than a feminine web of connection. In a hierarchical structure, the person who is alone at the top has the greatest autonomy. If one accepts hierarchical structure, it follows that autonomy decreases as one moves away from the top of the hierarchy. But Gilligan contends that women tend to value relationship and interaction rather than autonomous action and power. In Western philosophy, ethics has stressed autonomous decision-making and individual action rather than relationships, interaction, and cooperation. Thus, those who stress the need for autonomy in order to make moral decisions are following in the Western male philosophical tradition.

Following the emphasis on autonomy of traditional ethics, nurses would seem to lack power when they assume a wholistic stance. Consequently, those who emphasize autonomy often believe that it is desirable that nurses rid themselves of this role. But fostering the well-being of patients often requires nurses to work from a wholistic stance. In everyday nursing care, nurses have to facilitate the medical orders of physicians, utilize the facilities within the policies and procedures established by the institution or agency, and recognize the patient's wishes for a good life, as well as facilitate the nursing care that is their primary responsibility. These wholistic considerations are negative ones for nurses only from the point of view of hierarchical order. From Gilligan's interactive, democratic view, it is a highly valued position.

Wholistic care is a privileged stance from which to foster cooperative moral decisions by all involved. Difficult moral decisions should be made by teams involving the physician, nurse, patient, other professionals, representatives of the hospital, family, and, when available, an ethicist. Nurses are well situated to facilitate cooperative decision-making because they understand the medical position, the institution's vested interest and facilities, and usually the patient's and family's desires. Furthermore, a nurse is accustomed to making decisions that involve taking all of these various aspects into account.

The nurse, as an authority in nursing care, has his/her individual contributions and legitimate authority to contribute to this decision. When nurses make their primary stance gaining autonomy, they make sure that their position is heard and recognized above all others. Such assertions, although required at times, foster power struggles rather than cooperative decision-making. Nurses are uniquely situated to prevent power struggles. They have had to learn how to think from the other's position in order to work with physicians, administrators, patients, and families in planning everyday care. They have had to work within what Gilligan calls "the web of connection" (Gilligan, 1982, p. 62). This experience uniquely prepares them to help other health care professionals recognize that it is necessary to work within a web of connection to fulfill the moral imperative of health care. Such recognition will not come from militant demands for autonomy, but from helping others see that fostering the well-being of patients requires cooperative decision-making and action within a web of connection.

Unfortunately, most cases in ethics books involving cooperative decision-making concerning health care problems focus on making once-and-for-all judgments such as when to "pull the plug." In actual health care practice, moral judgments can rarely be made on a once-and-for-all basis. This is especially true for nurses because they work within a web of connection that requires constantly adjusting their care according to patient situations and the need to work with other health care professionals. Sometimes it becomes necessary for nurses to challenge the prescriptions, requirements, and desires of other team members while attempting to maintain the cooperative relationships necessary for patient care, as Margie Smith did so well.

THE MORAL IMPERATIVE TO REFORM HEALTH CARE

Cooperation and understanding are often not enough to ensure excellent nursing and patient care. Wholistic care and holistic care are both being threatened by current health care practice. The reduction in nursing staff and the added responsibility placed on nurses make it very difficult for nurses to work wholistically with others involved in health care and to care holistically for particular patients. When we first began interpreting nursing, we believed that nursing could be much improved by articulating the meaning of nursing as practiced and recognizing and realizing the inherent possibilities for more excellent practice. Nurses are now finding themselves in situations in which so many tasks are imposed on them and they have so little time with patients that it is difficult to pursue excellence. This situation indicates the soundness of those who have criticized us for assuming that nursing could be improved as it is currently practiced merely by disclosing its moral sense and its possibilities for excellence. We thought this approach would gradually expand the nurse's rightful authority to pursue excellent care. Today, it is evident that fostering excellence in nursing requires reform of health care.

Nurses need to critique health care practices, especially in hospitals, to disclose how nursing excellence is being sacrificed to corporate efficiency and the "bottom line." In our interpretation of nursing as practiced, we have attempted to show how critique can take place in nursing itself (Bishop & Scudder, 1990, 1991, 1996). This critique calls for nurses to create an alive and lively practice by pursuing the excellence in nursing that is possible in current practice. Nursing reform comes from recognition and realization of the possibilities for excellence that are inherent in the practice itself, but pursuit of excellence is being restricted by powerful agencies outside of nursing. Nurses have a moral obligation to reveal how these agencies are limiting patient care and to engage in actions that foster reform. This calls for critique and action as well as support and cooperation in wholistic care.

HOLISTIC CARE

Holistic care begins with the patient's first-person experience of illness and nursing care and the nurse's first-person experience of the practice of caring. It moves from this perspective to include scientific understanding, practical knowledge and skill, artistic and creative care, and recognition of nursing's moral sense. All of the foregoing are included in Claire Hastings' first-person account of her response to a person with arthritis for whom she holistically cared.

> I had a powerful clinical experience when I was working in the Rheumatology Screening Clinic. . . . An older woman in a wheelchair came with her daughter. I remember that she had terrible rheumatoid arthritis. When we say "terrible rheumatoid arthritis," we mean someone who might be presented in a textbook—one with a lot of deformities, who can't walk and is all twisted up and in pain. . . .
>
> When I see patients in this kind of situation, I usually begin by asking them some background questions about why they're here, what their history is, how long they've been ill, and so on. The first thing I asked her was whether she usually used a wheelchair. Was that the way she usually got around? And that question brought a flood of expression. Apparently, even though I thought her extremely disabled and deformed, this was the first time she had needed to use a wheelchair. She had somehow managed to cope with all the things that arthritis means, get around her house, take care of her family, and do her job, without having to resort to the symbolic state of "being in a wheel chair." Right away, that put us in touch with each other, and the encounter shifted to an emotional level. We were talking about feelings right from the beginning, before I had found out much about her.

It's hard to express, but there is a sense when you feel that you are making contact with the patient—and again I don't know whether it is the way you talk about the illness, the way you approach the patient, the kinds of questions you ask, or the language you use—but somehow, patients know that you know what they are talking about, that you have seen these kinds of things before. You understand *what they are*. You have dealt with the disease and the consequences of the illness daily, and you have a thorough knowledge of it. The illness is horrible to most people, and they never talk about it to the patient, but it is an everyday thing to you, something you have dealt with, something you know about, and therefore not horrendous or awful. I could feel that between us—that contact.

I then moved into doing a physical assessment and looking at her various joints. Thinking about this later, I realized one of the ways I was able to communicate with her, really get to some of the things she felt, was just by the way I looked at her joints. I made distinctions about swelling, the level of inflammation, and so on. It is possible to touch a person and move the person's hand or wrist , and say, "I can tell that this must be really painful right now," or "It looks like you haven't been able to use this hand for a long time.". . .

"Rheumatoid arthritis really has not been nice to you." She burst into tears, and her daughter did also, and I sat there, very close to losing it myself. She said: "You know, no one has ever talked about it as a personal thing before, no one's ever talked to me as if this were a thing that mattered, a personal event."*

Claire's holistic care begins by considering how arthritis has affected her patient's life. Thus, her care concentrates first on illness before moving to disease. Illness, according to Tristram Engelhardt, is what is experienced by a person who becomes a patient while disease is the pathological definition of that illness used in diagnosis by physicians (Engelhardt, 1982, p. 142). Illness, according to Mary Rawlinson, "names that experience in which our own everyday embodied capacities fail us. Illness obstructs our ordinary access to the world and presents the body as a signifier for the way in which we are limited and can be impeded in our encounter with the world" (Rawlinson, 1982, p. 75). Claire empathetically recognizes how arthritis has limited her patient's life and how valiantly she has struggled to maintain aspects of her former life by sharing in the care of home and family. Now she faces a further shrinking of her world by being confined to a wheelchair. When her patient acknowledges that "no one has ever talked about it as a personal thing before, no one's ever talked to me as if this were a thing that mattered, a personal event," she is not merely referring to Claire's comment about rheumatoid arthritis not being kind to her. In-

---

*From *The Primacy of Caring: Stress and Coping in Health and Disease* (pp. 9–11) by Patricia Benner and Judith Wrubel, 1989, Menlo Park, CA: Addison-Wesley. Used with permission.

stead, she is referring to the sensitive way in which Claire has appreciatively acknowledged how her illness has limited her lived world and is now threatening to further shrink it.

Although Claire's holistic care begins with illness, it also includes scientific knowledge of arthritis. In fact, she describes a textbook example. In examining the patient's joints, however, she uses her practical knowledge of how arthritis affects patients, gained from other nurses and her years of thoughtful practice. She synthesizes both theoretical and practical understanding of arthritis and the lived world of her patient in a way that assures her patient that she really cares for her as a person. Claire's care is personal in that she responds personally to the person she encounters. Her care is artful in the sensitive way she moves the patient's joints, responds to the patient's feelings, and communicates her feelings to the patient. A strong moral sense pervades her care. The plight of her patient calls her to nursing care. She is not *the* nurse, performing a professionally dictated activity: she is called to care personally as well as professionally for this person suffering from "terrible" arthritis.

Claire's holistic care includes the bio-psycho-social interpretation of holistic care. But scientific interpretations of biology, psychology, and sociology are only one source of the meaning of her care. She does not convert these sciences to applied sciences that prescribe nursing practice in a way that devalues the skills and understanding gained from the practice of nursing. The personal and spiritual dimensions of her care are not add-on components of her practice, but are integral aspects of her holistic care.

Claire's holistic care includes personal, esthetic, and moral care—dimensions of being that are usually considered spiritual. These ways-of-being include value dimensions of holistic nursing that are excluded from the sciences by their very nature. The spiritual is not an add-on dimension to the bio-psycho-social approach. Instead, it is an integral dimension of holistic care that gives new meaning to holistic nursing.

Spiritual meaning concerns a very different kind of meaning from that of the sciences. According to Huston Smith (1965), there are two fundamental meanings of meaning. The first is the most common usage. This is what we refer to when we ask someone, "What does this word mean?" The meaning we ask for can come from everyday language or from some theoretical treatment of the world, such as biological, psychological, or sociological systems of meaning. The other meaning has to do with the fundamental worth of our lives. This spiritual meaning is what we seek when we ask, "Does life really have any meaning?" We are asking, "Does life have a value or worth beyond its biological, psychological, or sociological meaning?" In nursing, this raises such questions as "Why should we buck the system to ensure better care?" "Should we use every possible means to keep persons alive who are suffering pain with no hope of recovery?" "Why should my care strive to reach beyond minimal professionally prescribed care to become excellent personal, creative care?"

The importance of spiritual meaning for nursing becomes evident in Viktor Frankl's (1962) interpretation of the meaning of life. Frankl was a Jewish psychiatrist who survived the worst of the concentration camps during the Holocaust. He soon recognized that what he had been taught about human beings in psychology did not account for why some survived and others did not. He discovered that those who survived did so because their life had a spiritual meaning that gave them the power to persist and to struggle. According to Paul Tillich (1952), the fundamental struggle of modern life is to find spiritual meaning adequate to give persons the courage to be.

Holistic care helps patients recover the spiritual meaning that fuels the courage to be in the face of illness and death. When patients confront serious illness, they often lose the deep sense of meaning that formerly gave them the courage to be. A patient who had formerly been a crusading, outgoing judge, when faced with his imminent death, retreated from life. He had cared for his family, clients, and others but, in the face of death, simply gave up. When confronted with how his retreat from life was affecting his family, he responded straightforwardly, "I gotcha." (Cousins, 1989, p. 24) Then he began to eat normally, play bridge, take walks, chat with other patients, follow the news, and most importantly, to communicate with his wife and his sons. The judge's recovery of the courage to be shows why holistic care includes a deeper source of meaning than merely staying alive.

> It was a magnificent example of how the human spirit could make a difference—not just in prolonging one's life but in bolstering the lives of others. The judge's deep sense of purpose didn't reverse the disease—the cancer had spread so widely to the vital organs that it was only a question of time before it would claim his life. But he was able to govern the circumstances of his passing in a way that provided spiritual nourishment to the people who loved him. He died in character. This was his gift to everyone who knew him.*

At the end, the judge recovered the spirit that had empowered his life. That spirit cannot be neatly placed in the category of the spiritual in parallel with the biological, sociological, and psychological. The spiritual names that deep meaning that calls forth the courage to be in the face of death and illness.

When a patient's courage to be is threatened by death and illness, the routine treatment of the nurse is inadequate. Such situations call for holistic care. Holistic care affirms the worth of persons who suffer illness and debilitation by seeking to understand and empathize with their lived world. Holistic care integrates objective scientific knowledge with the understanding and skills of the practice of nursing and incorporates these unified theoretical ways of care into the lived world of patients and nurses. The lived world, unlike the objective, theoretical world, is embued with esthetic, moral, and personal meanings. Holistic care embodies these meanings as an integral aspect of, rather than as additions to, nursing care. When nursing is holistic, the spiritual meaning of nursing care evokes the courage to be an excellent nurse who encourages and empowers patients to live as well as possible in their world.

---

*From *head first-the biology of hope*, by Norman Cousins, 1989. Used by permission of Dutten, a division of Pengum Putnam, Inc.

Study Questions

1. What is the difference between *wholistic* and *holistic* care?
2. Why do Anne and Jack believe that wholistic care is essential for patient well-being? Do you believe that nurses should be primarily responsible for wholistic care? Why or why not?
3. Evaluate Margie Smith's care of Mrs. Cooper as an exemplar of wholistic care and holistic care.
4. Anne and Jack contend that Margie's care follows Gilligan's interpretation of caring through a web of connection. After reading this chapter, do you think they interpret Margie's care correctly? After giving your answer, turn to Chapter 7 and participate in the dialogue between Jack and Anne concerning the issue of advocating patients rights and care in a web of connection.
5. What dimensions of holistic care does Claire Hastings' care of the arthritic patient add to Margie Smith's care of Mrs. Cooper?
6. What are the two fundamental meanings of meaning, according to Huston Smith, and how are they involved in holistic care?
7. Why do Anne and Jack believe that the spiritual concerns a different dimension of meaning from the biological, psychological, and sociological meanings?
8. What do Viktor Frankl and Paul Tillich contribute to the meaning of holistic care?
9. Discuss the judge's struggle to find the courage to be as an exemplar of the spiritual in holistic care. How could a nurse have assisted him in his struggle?
10. Critique the last paragraph of the chapter as a summary of holistic care. Do you believe that it should have included wholistic care? Why or why not?
11. Reform of health care as it relates to nurses can take the form of collective action or individual action. Cases 21 and 67 in Fry & Veatch are examples of each type of reform. In Case 21, Mrs. Tomlinson faces a difficult decision concerning whether to support collective action to improve nursing. What choice would you have made and why? Do you believe that collective action is an effective and moral means of improving nursing? In Case 67, Sandy Bardenilla faces the issue of whistle-blowing in a case involving questionable actions by physicians that were not challenged by the hospital. Do you think individual attempts at reform are needed? In what ways did her attempt at reform go beyond whistle-blowing?

References

Benner, Patricia, & Wrubel, Judith. (1989). *The primacy of caring: Stress and coping in health and disease*. Menlo Park, CA.: Addison-Wesley.

Bishop, Anne H., & Scudder, John R., Jr. (1990). *The practical, moral, and personal sense of nursing: A phenomenological philosophy of practice*. Albany, NY: State University of New York Press.

Bishop, Anne H., & Scudder, John R., Jr. (1991). *Nursing: The practice of caring*. New York: National League for Nursing, Jones and Bartlett.

Bishop, Anne H., & Scudder, John R., Jr. (1996). *Nursing ethics: Therapeutic caring presence*. Sudbury, MA: Jones and Bartlett.

Bishop, Anne H., & Scudder, John R., Jr. A phenomenological interpretation of holistic nursing. *Journal of Holistic Nursing*, 15, (2) pp. 103–111.

Cousins, Norman. (1989). *Head first: The biology of hope*. New York: E. P. Dutton.

Englehardt, H. Tristram, Jr. (1982) Illnesses, diseases, and sicknesses. In *The Humanity of the Ill*. ed. Victor Kestenbaum. Knoxville: University of Tennessee Press. (pp. 142–156).

Frankl, Viktor. (1962). *Man's search for meaning: An introduction to logotherapy*. New York: Simon and Schuster.

Fry, S. T. and Veatch, R. M. (2000). *Case Studies in Nursing Ethics 2nd edition*. Boston, MA. Jones & Bartlett.

Gilligan, Carol. (1982). *In a different voice. Psychological theory and women's development*. Cambridge, MA: Harvard University Press.

Rawlinson, Mary C. (1982). Medicine's discourse and the practice of medicine. In Victor Kestenbaum (Ed.), *The humanity of the ill*. (pp. 69–85). Knoxville: University of Tennessee Press.

Smith, Huston. (1965). *Condemned to meaning*. New York: Harper & Row.

Smith, Margie. (1993). Two legs to stand on. *American Journal of Nursing*, 93:12, pp. 43–44.

Tillich, Paul. (1952). *The courage to be*. New Haven, CT: Yale University Press.

Chapter

Caring Presence

Holistic care by nurses is experienced by patients as caring presence. Caring presence is often lacking in health care. Richard Zaner (1985) points out that patients want to know that those "who are taking care of them *really* care" for them (p. 92). This statement implies that patients more often receive effective and efficient care than they encounter caring presence. Roberta Messner (1993) reports that many studies of patient satisfaction have revealed that "patients' unmet expectations rarely have to do with competence. More often the problem is a perception of insensitivity to their needs or lack of respect for their viewpoint—in a word, caring" (p. 38).

Caring presence does not mean an emotive, sentimental, or maudlin expression of feeling toward patients. It is a personal presence that assures others of another's concern for their well-being. This way-of-being fosters trust, mutual concern, and positive attitudes that promote good health. When caring presence pervades a health care setting, the whole atmosphere of that setting is transformed so that not only is sound therapy fostered, but patients appreciate, take pride in, and feel part of the health care endeavor. The appreciation of many patients for the caring presence that pervades a free clinic was expressed in a note to the staff.

> . . . you are so much a part of all of our lives. You give so much and ask so little in return. During our lifetime we are touched by many people that criss-cross our lives. But we are indeed blessed when the most caring, loving people with so much compassion in their hearts touch our hearts and life and are always there for you. Because of you very beautiful people you have made our community a better place to live.

Caring presence also supports patients facing anxiety, suffering, and death. No one ought to face pain, uncertainty, or death alone and unsupported. When patients are not supported by family and friends, nurses often offer them the support and companionship they need. For example, nurses ensured that a very young child who had lived his entire life in the hospital was not left alone.

> As the parents had become gradually less and less involved, quite naturally those who were with Johnny most often and most intimately, especially the primary-care nurses, had effectively bonded with him, to the point that they seemed even to resent the parents and took the parents' apparent lack of concern quite personally. Even the attending [physician] seemed bound up with the child in a more personal way than I had witnessed before. "Taking care of" Johnny had shifted into "caring for" Johnny. (Zaner, 1993, p. 42)

Most people are not so alone. Many have an abundance of relatives and friends who support them with caring presence. But nurses are with patients in ways and situations that visitations to hospitals do not allow, and they have knowledge and expertise in relating to the patients that visitors do not possess. For example, a popular retired librarian was being visited in the hospital by another librarian and a fellow church member. When her visitors arrived, they found a woman sitting in the room who informed them that their friend was in the bathroom. Then she explained that she had been the librarian's nurse for a considerable period of time, but had been transferred to another unit. She knew that this patient was anxious because doctors had been unable to find out the cause of her illness. The nurse had dropped by to inquire about her progress and to give her support. After the patient returned and the nurse had left, the patient related how this nurse's caring presence had helped her live with the anxiety of being seriously ill without knowing why.

Caring presence often fosters the healing process itself. It often directly transforms the patient. Encountering caring presence fosters the well-being of patients by transforming their way-of-being in the world. When giving an injection, a reassuring nurse lessens the anxiety of the patient and thus the tenseness in the muscles, thereby making the injection less painful. In most therapeutic care, the reduction of tension and anxiety fosters healing and well-being.

The degree to which caring presence directly fosters healing has been highly problematic in health care literature. However, the work of Norman Cousins (1989) with physicians and nurses and the work of Delores Kreiger (1981) and Janet Quinn (1981) with nurses in therapeutic touch indicates that caring relationships can directly foster healing. Regardless of the degree to which healing is fostered directly by caring presence, caring presence supports patients in the way implied by Gilligan's interpretation of caring as "an activity of relationship, of seeing and responding to need, taking care of the world by sustaining the web of connection so that no one is left alone" (Gilligan, 1982, p. 62). Not being left alone requires more than simply being attended to. It requires the personal presence of others. Thus, it affirms Zaner's contention that patients not only want to be cared for, but they want to know that those who care for them truly care (Zaner, 1985, p. 96).

Obviously, caring presence is much needed in nursing, but caring presence requires fuller articulation than we have given. Our articulation will include descriptions of personal relationships, of caring, and of presence. We will attempt this articulation assisted by the work of Martin Buber (1970), Nel Noddings (1984), and Richard Zaner (1981).

BUBER: PERSONAL RELATIONS

Buber (1970) described two ways-of-being with others that are especially appropriate to human relationships in nursing. He contrasted personal I-*Thou* relationships with impersonal I-*It* relationships. The following example illustrates both relationships.

> Sarah is a 38-year-old woman with lymphoma. She has two young daughters, aged 3 and 5. She has been treated for over a year by an oncologist who often has difficulty developing personal relationships with his patients. However, Sarah's intelligence and interest in participating in the decisions regarding her care have fostered a personal relationship with the seemingly distant physician.
>
> The oncologist referred Sarah to a university medical center for a bone marrow biopsy. Securing bone marrow from Sarah in the past had proven extremely difficult because of her anatomy and bone structure. Sarah had agreed to go to the medical center because of its superior diagnostic equipment, but only on the condition that she would be given adequate pain medication.
>
> Due to some unfortunate circumstance, the physician who was to perform the biopsy was unable to do so, and after a long delay, a substitute was obtained. The substitute physician not only failed to respond to Sarah's request for more pain medication, but stopped Amy, the nurse, from getting the medication that had been ordered by the original physician to honor his prior agreement with Sarah. The substitute physician insisted on rigidly following what Sarah regarded as standardized procedures for any bone marrow biopsy. After several failed attempts to get bone marrow, another physician succeeded in getting some bone marrow with great difficulty. Both physicians conducted the biopsy with standard medication and procedures, paying no attention to Sarah's request for more pain medication. In contrast, Amy, assisting with the biopsy, listened attentively to Sarah's request and the reasons for making that request. Sarah later commented that Amy was the only sensible (and sensitive) member of the biopsy team and vowed never to return to that hospital again.
>
> After the biopsy, Sarah's husband commented to Amy that his wife had incredible strength. The nurse expressed her agreement, having cared for Sarah during the trying, painful procedure. But the physicians who had performed the operation responded to the husband's

comment with ironic disdain. They had encountered the patient as being an uncooperative patient who overreacted to pain and tried to tell them how to conduct the biopsy.

The physicians related to this patient as an It—a thing to be put in the category of "uncooperative patient" because she did not respond to their standardized treatment in ways that facilitated the biopsy. In contrast, Amy responded to Sarah personally as Thou. During the biopsy, she had come to know Sarah as an intelligent person who attempted to make the best of a difficult situation made worse by insensitive physicians. In her brief relationship with Sarah, Amy had encountered the same person the husband knew from sharing her long and difficult struggle with cancer.

In this example, incompetent behavior should not be confused with impersonal behavior. During surgical procedures, competent physicians use information concerning the patient obtained from charts and interviews. Such competency does not constitute a personal relationship with the patient. Amy secured the agreed-on pain medication by following medical orders on the chart, but her assessment of the situation came from relating to Sarah in a mutually responsive way that took seriously her patient's right to insist that the physicians give the pain medication previously agreed on and prescribed for her particular situation.

All health care workers are well aware that patients often make inappropriate suggestions about their care. Professionals are experts concerning what is best for *the patient*. But in the foregoing case, the biopsy was not done to *the patient*, but to a particular person who, by working with her regular oncologist, had come to sound conclusions concerning her response to pain and the resistance of her bone structure. Although her oncologist was known for his difficulty relating to persons, he had been able to relate to Sarah personally in matters concerning her situation and treatment. The oncologist knew more than she did about cancer and treatment. But she had learned much from him in their relationship of mutual respect and shared concern for her well-being. Although during the operation Amy was much more personable than Sarah's oncologist, they both related to Sarah as Thou.

In the preceding case, both the nurse and the oncologist are in I-Thou relationships with Sarah. I-Thou relationships concern a way-of-being with another person. Neither the style nor the length of the relationship is relevant. For example, Amy is personable; the oncologist is not. Amy has known the patient only a short time, whereas the oncologist has known her for about a year. But in each case, Sarah is related to as a person and is responded to as she is present. Sarah is a full partner in the relationship in that she is listened to and included in decisions about her ongoing treatment. This mutual relationship of personal response to each other is essential to all I-Thou relationships. In I-Thou relationships, both partners recognize the right of each other to his/her way of being. In I-Thou relationships, whole persons encounter each other as beings who are present to each other. Sarah related to both her physician and nurse as persons, albeit persons with special knowledge and skills encountered in special relationships. Buber recognized that, due to this imbalance, therapeutic relationships cannot be fully mutual ones, and therefore they constitute a special form of I-Thou relationships. In Sarah's relationships with her nurse and oncologist, the mutuality of their relationship is asymmetrical; nevertheless, they respond to each other as the whole person who is present in their encounter.

In contrast to the I-Thou relationship between Sarah and her oncologist and nurse, her relationship to the physicians who performed the biopsy was an I-It relationship. Instead of responding to her as a person, the physicians regarded her as *the* patient from whom bone marrow was to be taken. She was an uncooperative patient in that she insisted on more pain medication, thereby implicitly questioning the physicians' judgment. The physicians' knowledge about biopsies and human anatomy dictated their treatment of the patient, without regard to her response to their treatment. They seemed in no way present to her suffering presence. For Buber, I-It relationships are characterized by detachment from the other, by use of knowledge about the other to categorize the other and to treat the other in a standard way, and by objectification of the otherness of the other. In an I-It relationship, the mutuality and recognition of the other that arise from reciprocal presence and personal response are absent.

Most nurses readily recognize I-It relationships between physicians and patients and obvious I-It relationships in nurse-patient relationships. Buber's description of I-It relationships can help nurses recognize less obvious I-It relationships in nursing, such as professionally and technically defined relationships. In I-It relationships, one person detaches himself/herself from another in order to gain knowledge that makes it possible to control the other or, in professional language, to intervene in the life of the other. In the professional model, the nurse detaches himself/herself from the patient to consider what any competent nurse would do in these circumstances. Knowledge of good nursing comes primarily from education and is condensed in the form of maxims to be applied in situations: "in situation x the nurse does y." In this scenario, the good patient is compliant and follows the dictates of the professional nurse. The client is not present as a person but only as *the* client to be controlled by the maxims of the profession.

The technical interpretation of nursing is even more aptly described by Buber's treatment of I-It than is the professional interpretation. In the technical interpretation, the nurse is supposed to remain detached from the patient in order to meet the requirements of science. The nurse is to use knowledge obtained from scientific study to categorize and prescribe interventions to alter the patient's behavior. The patient is dealt with as an example of x to be treated by y, but not as a person.

In the preceding discussion, we have treated I-It relationships in nursing that tend to blind nurses to the moral and personal sense of nursing. Our treatment of these I-It relationships should not lead to the conclusion that all

I-It relationships are to be avoided. There are many situations that call for I-It relationships. Buber, in fact, contended that it is impossible to continually remain in I-Thou relationships without being "consumed" (Buber, 1970, p. 85). It may also be desirable to be in an I-It relationship to perform certain functions. Technological functions in nursing practice often require that nurses temporarily forget the person and focus on the function. This way of placing nurses in I-It relationships with patients does not mean that nurses should forget that they are working with and on fellow human beings. A way of recognizing the rights of persons in I-It relationships is needed. Buber does not give us this way, but his description of I-It and I-Thou relationships does help nurses to distinguish between the personal and the impersonal and to recognize how the impersonal can subvert the moral sense of nursing.

I-It (Thou) Relationships

A way is needed to describe impersonal relationships that supports the moral and personal sense of nursing. Sally Gadow (1985) makes evident the need for such a relationship in her contention that nurses need to attend to the body object without reducing the patient to the moral status of an object (pp. 32–33). A relationship that makes it possible to deal with other persons objectively while recognizing their inherent dignity and worth has been described as an I-It (T*hou*) relationship (Scudder & Mickunas, 1985). For example, a nurse searching for a vein in an arm scarred by repeated intravenous injections and weakened by chemotherapy needs to temporarily focus on the function rather than on the worried, suffering patient. By focusing on the function, this nurse would foster the patient's well-being by ensuring a successful procedure with minimal harm. But when focusing on the function, he/she should not forget that the patient is a person, as the parenthetical T*hou* indicates. I-It (Thou) describes a relationship in which a nurse can attend to the body object technically and professionally without reducing the patient to the moral status of an object.

I-It (Thou) relationships require recognition of patient rights. If a patient screams "Stop! You're killing me!" a nurse might stop, reasoning, "This is a fellow human being who has the right to decide how much pain to endure." Rights arguments are impersonal. A person has rights as a citizen, a patient, a nurse, and ultimately as a human being. Rights are granted to individuals by impersonally placing them in categories. Being placed in the category of patient implies equal but not uniform treatment. Patients, like all human beings, are unique individuals who have a right to be treated individually. As Buber (1958) has pointed out, individuality refers to I-It relationships because individuality is determined by comparing one person with another (p. 62). For example, the patient in the bone marrow example is different from most patients in being more susceptible to pain and having harder, thicker bones. By emphasizing this difference, the nurse in that example could have argued with the physicians for individualized treatment for her patient. In so doing, she would argue impersonally for individualized treatment on the grounds that her patient is a human being and therefore has the right to individualized treatment like any other human being.

When nurses are in I-It (Thou) relationships with patients, they not only recognize patient rights, but also are open to the possibility of entering into personal relationships with patients. The parentheses enclosing the word T*hou* indicate that the nurse maintains an awareness that this is a person, even when treating the patient impersonally. This awareness fosters the movement from the impersonal to the personal. For example, imagine that Amy is intent on treating and bandaging Sarah's wound when suddenly Sarah asks her, "How can I tell my young children that I am dying?" This calls for transition from an I-It relationship to an I-Thou relationship. It is possible that Amy might have no better answer to the question posed than Sarah; nevertheless, she should respond personally to this invitation to dialogue by entering her patient's intimate life. Her response could eventually lead her into a relationship of caring presence with a dying person—a personal relationship that one nurse has called the most fulfilling in her career (Bishop & Scudder, 1990, pp. 95–96).

TRIADIC DIALOGUE

As important as personal relationships are in nursing care, they are not the end of nursing care. Nursing care is a relationship designed to foster the well-being of the patient. One problem in interpreting nursing relationships as I-Thou relationships is that I-T*hou* describes a personal relationship with no end beyond itself, such as friendship. But nursing has an end beyond the relationship itself. Nurse-patient relationships are established to foster the well-being of one of the partners, called the *patient* or the *client*. The nurse-patient relationship is not created to develop deep personal relationships, but to foster the healing and health of the patient.

Fostering the well-being of patients (the moral sense of nursing) can be included in the nurse-patient relationship through *triadic dialogue* (Bishop & Scudder, 1990). In triadic dialogue, nurse and patient respond to each other as persons for the purpose of fostering the well-being of the patient. Triadic dialogue occurred between nurse and patient in the episode described in chapter two.

> She had a special way of offering her help in concrete ways like washing my back and my feet, which I literally could not reach that morning. "I suggest that you . . .," and "what you could do is turning your body . . .," yes she was assisting me, never taking over. I was in command, I felt. I mattered. Even though the only thing I could manage was steering the shower handle. (Harder, 1993, p. 172)

The dialogue between the nurse and patient is tactile as well as verbal. The nurse's way of washing the patient assures the patient that eventually she will be able to wash herself, and the nurse's speech suggests how the patient can begin to bathe herself. Amazingly, this is done with such sensitivity and artistry that the patient feels she is "in command," even though she is only capable of manipulating the shower handle. Even though the nurse is actually bathing the patient, the patient is already beginning self-care.

This nurse's care of the patient is an excellent example of what Martin Heidegger (1962) has called *authentic care*. Authentic care empowers patients to care for themselves. In contrast, *dependent care* (our term rather than Heidegger's) takes care away from patients by making them dependent on the caregiver (Scudder, 1990). Unfortunately, the term *caring presence* often connotes dependent care. But authentic caring presence empowers persons to care for themselves as much as possible.

Triadic dialogue is uniquely structured to foster authentic care. In contrast to dyadic dialogue, which focuses on the relationship of the partners and on sharing between the partners, triadic dialogue calls for fostering the well-being of one of the partners through empowerment of that partner in an I-Thou relationship. In the foregoing example, the nurse and the patient are in an I-Thou relationship that is focused on fostering the well-being of the patient by bathing her in a way that teaches, encourages, and empowers her to bathe herself in the future.

Noddings: Caring

Nurses foster the well-being of patients through caring relationships. The description of caring by Noddings is especially appropriate to an interpretation of caring presence. Noddings assumes that personal relationships are "ontologically basic and the caring relation" is "ethically basic" (Noddings, 1984, p. 150). These assumptions support the primacy of personal relationships in Buber's thought and the moral sense of those relationships in triadic dialogue.

Noddings describes caring in a way that makes its moral sense evident. The essential elements in a caring relationship include "*engrossment* and *motivational displacement* on the part of the one-caring and a form of *responsiveness* or *reciprocity* on the part of the cared-for" (Noddings, 1984, p. 150). According to Noddings, the one-caring is first engrossed in the other's life and then shifts motivational concern from self to the other. She contends that when I am engrossed, "I receive the other into myself, and I see and feel with the other" (p. 30). Thus, caring involves attempting to experience the world as the other experiences it by seeing through "the eyes of the cared-for" (p. 13). For example, Amy became engrossed in Sarah's situation and was able to become present to her suffering. In contrast, the physicians were preoccupied with completing a biopsy by following routine procedures. In addition, they seemed preoccupied with their own well-being and not with that of the patient. One physician even complained to the patient during the biopsy that he would not get paid for his services.

The motivational shift from the well-being of the one-caring to the one-cared-for is the other essential ingredient in care, as described by Noddings. In this shift, there is "displacement of interest from my own reality to the reality of the other" so that I "see the other's reality as a possibility for my own" (p. 14). The other's possibility is fostered by taking "special regard for the particular person in a concrete situation" (p. 24). Amy made that motivational shift to the well-being of Sarah in her concrete situation. In contrast, the physicians in this case were not engaged in care for this patient; instead, they were carrying out prescribed procedures for any patient. Although the nurse's care involved professional procedures, her way-of-being with the patient was not primarily a professional one but a human one of caring presence.

In caring relationships, as described by Noddings, the one-cared-for responds to care by appreciation for care given or by going on with his/her life in the way that care has made possible. Sarah and her husband greatly appreciated the care Amy provided, especially since it was present in such difficult circumstances. This appreciation was deeply felt even though Amy was not in a position to change the way that the procedure was conducted. Mrs. Cooper exemplifies another response to care received by taking up her life in the way that Margie's care made possible. She reveals how this care has enhanced her life by visiting Margie with her grandchildren "in tow."

In addition to describing care as engrossment, motivational shift, and patient response, Noddings makes a distinction between natural caring and ethical caring that is significant for nursing practice and especially for nursing ethics. Natural caring is "that relationship in which we respond as one-caring out of love or natural inclination" (Noddings, 1984, p. 5). We enter into a relationship of natural caring when "we accept the natural impulse to act on behalf of the present other" (p. 83). Presumably, the nursing scholar we referred to earlier who remarked that nurses feel guilty when we point out the moral sense of nursing meant that nurses cannot always operate on the basis of natural caring and therefore feel that they are neglecting the moral sense. Nurses cannot always—and perhaps cannot usually—act out of natural caring. This dilemma of having to care in the absence of natural caring can be resolved through Noddings's distinction between natural caring and ethical caring. Noddings contends that even when we are not motivated by natural caring, we can care because we want to be a caring person. The desire to be a caring person is motivated and empowered by appreciative remembrance of having been cared for by others.

When ethical caring is applied to nursing, nurses would care out of the desire to be caring nurses rather than out of natural care. But does this not assign a higher priority to caring out of a desire to be a caring nurse than to caring naturally? It would do so for nurses for whom caring merely means following the prescriptive maxim that "Good nurses care." However, if nursing is essentially caring, then being a caring nurse requires placing caring for patients above other values in practice. In nursing practice, however, being a caring nurse and valuing caring are so integrally related that such separation would be artificial and lead to inauthentic nursing. When nurses are motivated by ethical caring, they do what they do because they value caring for persons, even those persons for whom they do not naturally care. For example, when a nurse does not naturally care for an obnoxious patient, he/she would care for that patient out of the desire to be a caring person but one who cares in the way that nurses care.

Although Noddings's interpretation of caring contributes much to the understanding of nursing care, it should be tested by being placed in the context of nursing practice. Placing it in this context will show that her interpretation of care needs to include natural caring in the ethical, consider competing moral desires and limited time, and recognize the caring in practice.

NATURAL CARING IN THE ETHICAL

Noddings reserves the term *ethical* for caring that is done out of the desire to be a caring person rather than out of natural caring. She makes clear that ethical caring does not have a higher priority than natural caring. For her, natural caring is preferable to ethical caring. The implication of this interpretation of caring for nursing is that nurses should care naturally when possible, but when natural care is not possible, then they should care ethically. For example, a nurse who does not naturally care for a difficult patient would do so because he/she wants to be a caring nurse. But to be caring, the nurse would have to become engrossed in the patient's situation and shift concern from self to the patient. Because this shift gives priority to the well-being of the patient, the nurse cannot become a caring nurse by *seeking* to be a caring nurse, but only by seeking the well-being of clients. Consequently, desiring to be a caring nurse may initiate care for the other, but a nurse is a caring nurse only when he/she attempts to foster the well-being of others, thus fulfilling the moral sense of nursing.

One interpretation of Noddings eliminates the shift from self (I want to be a caring person) to actual caring (being engrossed in and acting to promote another's well-being). Although Noddings argues that in ethical caring, I care because I want to be a good person, she also asserts that ethical caring arises out of valuing caring itself. Ethical caring arises from "an evaluation of the caring relationship as good, as better than, superior to, other forms of relatedness. . . . The source of my obligation [to care] is the value I place on the relatedness of caring" (Noddings, pp. 83–84). Here Noddings seems to say that I want to be a caring person because I recognize the worth of caring relationships. But even so, to enter into a caring relationship, I would have to refocus my attention and effort from the worth of caring to engrossment with and actual care for the person who needed my care.

Interpreting ethical caring as caring done out of recognition of the worth of caring rather than only out of the desire to be a caring person makes ethical caring less egocentric. But it does not explain why caring out of natural care is not designated ethical caring, while caring out of recognition for the worth of care, and hence the desire to be a caring person, is designated as ethical. Noddings's reasoning may be that, if I care for someone because I desire to, then my action has no ethical merit. However, if I care for someone because I value caring and therefore want to be a caring person in opposition to my natural inclinations, then my actions are virtuous or meritorious. She contends that when the remembrance of having been cared for "sweeps over us as a feeling—as an 'I must'—in response to the plight of the other," it encounters a "conflicting desire to serve our own interests" (Noddings, 1984, pp. 79–80). Since ethical caring is marked by conflicting desires, it "requires an effort that is not needed in natural caring" (p. 80). Therefore, in order to be ethical, according to Noddings, I must choose to act against my natural inclinations by caring for those I do not naturally care for because I value caring.

Noddings seems to believe that an action can be designated as ethical only when a person is forced to choose to act morally against natural desires. Hence, for Noddings, acting out of natural caring cannot be called ethical. This reasoning could lead to the odd conclusion that nurses can be ethical only when they do not care naturally for any of their patients. We can escape this outlandish conclusion by interpreting the ethical to include actions done out of both natural caring and out of the desire to be a caring person. Thus, nursing ethics would include fostering the well-being of clients out of natural caring as well as out of the desire to be a caring nurse.

CONFLICTING MORAL DESIRES AND LIMITED TIME

Why inclusion of natural caring in the ethical is appropriate in nursing can be shown by considering dilemmas nurses face that fall outside of the context of Noddings's natural caring versus ethical caring. In contending that ethical caring "requires an effort that is not needed in natural caring" (p. 80), Noddings fails to consider moral tensions faced in natural caring that require considerable moral effort. One such effort occurs when nurses, in natural caring, find themselves torn between care for patient and self. For instance, a nurse completing an understaffed night shift, her body aching and exhausted and her nerves on edge, may feel a natural desire to care for a patient who especially needs her care. The nurse faces a moral choice between a natural desire to care for the patient and a natural desire to care for self. It took Nurse Echo Heron many exhausting years filled with tension to learn that those who care for others must also care for themselves (Heron, 1987).

In nursing practice, nurses can and often do naturally care for persons in circumstances that force them to make moral choices due to limited time. For example, at the end of his/her shift, a nurse faces several situations involving natural caring. One patient, who is several hours post-operative, needs to be catheterized; another patient is experiencing severe post-operative pain with no post-operative orders; a third is anxious about going home because no one is at home to help her after discharge. The nurse naturally cares for each of these persons; he/she would like to care for each of them. Unfortunately, time to care for all three is lacking. The nurse is faced with choosing between the urgent need to catheterize and to get an order for pain medication and the need to counsel a patient with whom he/she has developed a special relationship. The nurse reasons that the next nurse probably would not have the special relationship, but could complete the catheterization and call the physician for the order for pain medication. Requiring the first two patients to wait, however, would prolong their suffering. We give this example to show that moral dilemmas in nursing are not limited to situations in which the alternative is between natural care and ethical care, and to illustrate that moral choice is needed when nurses care for different patients out of natural caring but have limited time. The pressure of time is almost always present in concrete moral situations, but is often ignored in abstract discussions of moral decision-making.

Those who care for others often face the moral dilemma of choosing whom to care for, given limited time. For this reason, Martha Nussbaum writes that to "be a good human being is to have a kind of openness to the world.... a willingness to be exposed" (Moyers, 1989, p. 448). Nussbaum contends that good persons are open to and expose themselves to caring relationships, even knowing that they may be led to grief and tragedy as well as to fulfillment. Nussbaum claims that traditional ethics seeks to solve moral problems in a clear-cut and certain manner. Traditional ethics achieves its clarity and certainty by falsifying the complexity of moral situations (Nussbaum, 1986, pp. 343–372). Nurses are continually thrust into caring relationships in complex situations with time limitations that inherently involve both tragedy and fulfillment. Remaining open and exposed are moral imperatives for all who answer the call to care.

CARING IN PRACTICE

Noddings limits her treatment of caring to the subjective side of encounter with others. I care for others when I am engrossed in their situation and shift my concern from my well-being to their well-being. This shift of concern does require me to act. I "must act to eliminate the intolerable, to reduce the pain, to fill the need, to actualize the dream" (Noddings, 1984, p. 14). But in order to act to eliminate the intolerable, reduce the pain, fill the need, and actualize the dream, I need empowerment. In nursing, empowerment comes from appropriating the practice of nursing. When authentically appropriated, nursing practice becomes empowering possibilities rather than traditional directives. The practice of nursing empowers nurses to care, but it does not make choices concerning care for them.

Empowered action requires more than caring out of natural or ethical concern for the patient. The empowerment of nursing practice fits that aspect of being that Heidegger labeled "ready-to-hand," in that past practitioners have left us ways of caring for the ill and debilitated and of fostering healthy being. Nurses care for patients by appropriating these "ready" ways to care. That Noddings missed this aspect of care is evident in her treatment of practice in education, her field of expertise. For her, practice merely means learning how to care by doing it. She seems not to grasp the full meaning of practice, much less the significance of its inherent moral sense for ethics. For this reason, she does not call natural caring ethical.

If ethics in nursing concerns fulfilling its moral sense, then when the nurse acts to fulfill that sense, he/she is being moral whether acting out of natural caring or out of the desire to be a caring person. Natural caring appears to be more desirable than ethical caring because it directly fosters the well-being of the ill and debilitated rather than requiring a refocusing from desire to be a caring nurse or valuing caring itself to concern for the well-being of the patient. Ethical caring would seem to be supplementary to natural caring, in that it would come into play only when natural care is inadequate. Put positively, a morally good nurse would foster the well-being of patients as an act of natural caring whenever possible, but when a nurse does not care naturally, he/she would care because of ethical caring. Ethical caring would require a shift from valuing caring, and hence wanting to be a caring nurse, to concern for fostering the well-being of patients. This shift from self to other is called for by nursing practice—its inherent moral sense requires caring relationships that foster the well-being of others. Regardless of whether nurses care for patients naturally or out of the desire to be caring nurses, they should not separate the practice of caring from the subjective meaning of care. Separation of motive from action artificially separates care as concern from care as practice. Noddings's description of care as engrossment and motivational shift is an excellent description of the subjective experience of caring. This description does not refer to inner motivation that "causes" caring practice. It merely describes the subjective side of the integral relationship between care for patients (concern) and care of patients (practice).

The care *for* patients and the care *of* patients are integrally related in nursing practice. In a practice, meaning is implicit in doing. Consequently, subjective concern for patients often grows out of the experience of caring practice. The meaning of caring progressively informs practice as nurses learn care (concern) by engaging in caring (practice).

Learning meaning by participation in human activities is one of the primary ways that human beings learn. Remy Kwant (1965) describes how meaning develops in children in a way that suggests how the meaning of caring develops.

> We can verify all this when we observe how a child begins to act. He grows up in a house as in a little manipulable world, in which things are handled by the other occupants of the house. The child sees these

persons act and in their actions the meaning of the things is activated, brought to light. He begins to imitate and through imitation gradually makes his own the meaning which things have for the others. Thus he begins to act as a human being. The child sees in the actions of the others the realization of his own possibilities. In the same way he learns to speak. The child grows up in a speaking community. He imitates the sounds, appropriates the words and gradually begins to live in the meaning of these words. (Kwant, 1965, p. 81)

Noddings's belief that caring develops in the above manner is evident when she says, "I have a picture of those moments in which I was cared for and in which I cared, and I may reach toward this memory and guide my conduct by it" (Noddings, 1984, p. 80). For Noddings, becoming a caring presence depends on having experienced being cared for and of having cared for others.

Ways of caring are passed on to new generations through human habitation. Erazim Kohák (1984) explains how care is evident in human habitations.

It is a sense of a presence such as humans experience on entering a home in the dweller's absence. Unlike the abandoned, looted dwellings left in the wake of revolutions or the gutted shells of the inner city, . . . a dwelling, though empty, feels cared for, as if there were a cherishing and a rightness. The house *belongs*: on entering it, we sense its order not simply as an order, but specifically as the order of a *Lebenswelt*, of an inhabited context ordered by a caring presence. (p. 189)

In similar manner, the caring presence of those who have cared for the well-being of others before us inhabits the practice of nursing that we have inherited. We become nurses by inhabiting and appropriating their ways-of-being in our care for patients.

Nancy Diekelmann (1990) attempts to teach nurses the meaning of caring by engaging in dialogue with them concerning the meaning of their practice. She does not assume that they are already motivated to care and need only to learn how. Instead, Diekelmann attempts through dialogue to make evident the care (concern) that is inherently present in practice. The question about whether care (concern) comes prior to practice and motivates it, or comes out of the experience of caring (practice), is a major issue only to those who make the artificial separation of motive from action. To those who reject this artificial separation, it is enough to say that care (concern) and care (practice) are so integrally related to each other that it is impossible to say which comes first. It is possible, however, to identify engrossment and motivational shift as an integral aspect of nursing care. Patients refer to this subjective side of nursing care when they say that they want to know that the nurse who cares for them really cares for them. Engrossment and motivational shift are not experienced as something apart from practice, but in and through the practice of caring.

ZANER: CARING RESPONSE TO PRESENCE

Noddings's treatment of care and Zaner's treatment of presence (Zaner, 1981) can be formulated into an interpretation of caring presence especially significant for nursing ethics. Zaner places more emphasis on the response of others and on responsibility for others than does Noddings. Whereas Noddings focuses on describing the experience of the one caring as engrossment and motivational shift, Zaner focuses on describing the meeting of self and other as vivid presence and co-presence. In describing that meeting, he gives much more attention than Noddings to how the one-cared-for experiences the one-caring. In his description, the one-caring is experienced as available and empowering by the one-cared-for.

We will explore the meaning of caring presence by looking at it in light of Zaner's treatment of reflexive presence to the lived body, vivid presence, and co-presence. We say "in light of" his treatment because our purpose is not to fully explicate his treatment of these themes as they are developed in his book *The Context of Self* (1981). His treatment has generated our thought concerning caring presence and that thought has been further enhanced by personal dialogue with him concerning the meaning of presence and its implications for nursing ethics. Thus, Zaner's work has called forth a creative response from us. In response to Zaner, we first will show how Zaner's treatment of presence can enhance the understanding of nursing care. Then, by bringing Noddings's caring and Zaner's presence together, we will formulate a caring presence especially significant for nursing ethics.

REFLEXIVE PRESENCE TO THE LIVED BODY

Nursing requires care of the lived body. The relationship between nurse and patient is an unusual one in that two partners care for the lived body of one of them. Equally odd is that although patients live in their bodies, they may talk about them as if they were detached objects. They often need help from nurses to attend to and describe the experience of their lived bodies. In some cases, nurses even have to help patients learn how to live in their bodies again, as we will illustrate in a subsequent chapter.

One difficulty in appropriating Noddings's treatment of care for nursing is that it is so exclusively oriented to interpersonal care that it almost precludes focusing on care of the lived body. Zaner's treatment of reflexive presence helps remedy this deficiency. Zaner contends that as we engage the world we can be reflexively present to our own bodies. This reflexive presence is what makes it possible for us to know our bodies as lived. Most athletes, even though they are focused on the game, are aware of their bodies as they engage in sport. For example, a physician advised an overweight, sedentary patient to take up jogging. He warned the patient about overexerting his heart and gave him instructions concerning his target heart rate and how to check his pulse while jogging. The patient invited his brother, who was twenty years older than he but quite athletic, to run with him. The younger brother ran the mile faster than his older brother, but his heart rate did not return to normal within the expected time. In contrast, the older brother's heart rate returned to normal earlier than expected. When the younger brother asked his older brother, who was not a jogger, how he accomplished that, the older brother replied, "I listened to my body as I ran."

Most of us are not overtly conscious of our body as we live. One of the primary meanings of illness is that it forces us to attend to the lived body. We say, "My shoulder is stiff," "I can't get my breath," "My back aches," "I'm constipated." I pay no attention to my shoulder as I serve an ace past my tennis opponent. However, when my physician asks me if I have been short of breath, I respond, "Yes, in the third set in a match with an opponent half my age." "Bull!" my physician retorts, acknowledging that my lungs are functioning better than would be expected of someone my age. Because our shoulders and lungs go unnoticed until they trouble us, we have difficulty in describing our experience of them to nurses and physicians. When we attempt such description, we describe them in terms of our lived body and not of the body as an anatomical object. I say, "My shoulder is stiff," not "I have a torn rotator cuff"; or "I was out of breath after the first game of a very slow match," not "I am experiencing the onset of asthma." Once the asthma is diagnosed, however, I will be quite aware of the connection between my breathing and vigorous exercise. In fact, I may use it as an excuse for my inability to cover the court.

Nurses and physicians need to be able to draw out patients' experiences of their lived body. Unfortunately, physicians often—and nurses sometimes—request information about the body from patients in ways that lead patients away from their experience of their lived body. Often physicians are so focused on diagnosing disease that they carefully request experiences that will indicate the likelihood of a certain disease. Usually, some standard medical procedure based on theory controls what they ask for and what they attend to. Frequently, they dismiss unsolicited descriptions of the lived body of the patient as an irrelevant waste of their time.

The difference between using theoretical perspectives to select certain experiences of the body and eliciting the lived experience of a patient can best be shown by an example from clinical practice.

> Sam was a seventy-five-year-old man with a diagnosis of emphysema. He had been to his physician several times complaining of pain. When the physician asked him where the pain was located, he rubbed an area in his lower chest region, which the physician thought was due to Sam's chronic lung condition. Sam complained to a nurse one day that his pain was getting worse and that the physi-

cian did not seem to know what the problem was. The nurse asked Sam to show her just exactly where the pain was. When Sam pressed on the area of the pain, it was obviously not in the lung region but in the area just below the diaphragm, where Sam had a hernia from a previous surgery. The nurse asked him to describe in detail what the pain was like and how long he had had it. It seemed to the nurse that the pain as described was likely the result of a strangulated hernia. She suggested that Sam call his physician to discuss this possibility. Sam called the physician who arranged to see him almost immediately. Sam, however, had a coughing spell prior to seeing the physician, and the strangulation broke loose from the force of the cough. Almost immediately Sam's pain was relieved. When Sam's physician examined him, he confirmed that Sam's pain probably resulted from a strangulated hernia.

What the physician did not know was that his diagnosis was made possible by a nurse's caring presence to Sam's lived body rather than by medical preoccupation with symptoms that confirmed a previous diagnosis. Since nurses spend much more time than physicians with patients in on-going relationships, they have a special responsibility to help patients learn to be reflexively present to their own lived bodies. Such presence is necessary for patients to be able to assume responsibility for their own health care.

VIVID PRESENCE

In the preceding examples of care for Sam and Sarah, both nurses are obviously vividly present to their patients. Zaner (1981) describes vivid presence as a relationship in which persons are present to each other and at the same time aware of their shared presence. This shared presence is brought about by each of the partners "tuning in" to the other. This tuning in creates a shared common experience rather than "'two series of events,' yours and mine" (p. 230). In vivid presence, the partners create a common flow of experience in which each is aware of being in shared relationship.

> We, you and I, each in our own ways, *experience our relationship itself* ("we have a good marriage," or "we are really having fun," etc.), *as well as one another,* ("aren't you having a good time?") *and in the relationship, each relates himself to himself,* ("I'm having a good time!" "So am I!") *and to the other*" ("You didn't act like you were having a good time!" "Neither did you!"). (Zaner 1981, p. 231)

In vivid presence, we attune to each other in a way that leads us into a shared common experiencing of self in the world. The consciousness of each partner is focused on their shared world in which each person is reflexively aware of that person as being in the relationship.

In the foregoing description of vivid presence, Zaner is not focused on health care, but rather on how the self is constituted in relationships of vivid presence. We are interested in how vivid presence contributes to our understanding of nursing care. Consequently, our consideration of vivid presence will concern partners in asymmetrical relationships in which one partner is caring for the other while the other is receiving care. The implication of Zaner's vivid presence for nursing care can best be seen through an example from clinical practice. The following narrative was written by a nursing student working as a nurse extern.

> While working as a nurse extern one evening, I was checking on my patients' progress with dinner trays. In one lady's room, I casually asked how she was doing with her dinner tray. She stated, "Okay." We said a few words and as I was on my way out the door, she said she probably wasn't very hungry because her chest was "tight." I was busy but stopped in my tracks and asked her to tell me about this "tightness." The "tightness" turned out to be chest pain radiating to her left arm. I immediately told the charge nurse who called the physician who ordered oxygen and a medication. I stayed in the patient's room for forty-five minutes, monitoring her blood pressure every fifteen minutes. Suppose I hadn't asked another question?

In this example, the nurse and patient initially are not vividly present to each other. They share a casual, everyday experience of one helping the other in partaking of a meal. The presence becomes vivid when the nurse recognizes, in the patient's parting comment, an indication of impending danger. She returns to the patient, and they become vividly present to each other. The focus of their shared presence is one partner's consciousness of her body as she attempted to eat the meal. The nursing partner is able to elicit the patient's lived experience of her own body in a way that alerts the nurse to the possibility of a heart attack in progress. This occurs when the nurse shifts from the ordinary experience of helping with the meal to the vivid presence that elicited the patient's description of what she was experiencing in her own body. The patient is able to share that experience because her nurse helps her recover her reflexive presence of her body as she attempted to eat the meal. Through entering into a relationship of vivid caring presence with the patient, the nurse becomes aware of herself as a nurse—not as a student nurse extern, but as a *nurse* in the full meaning of that term.

In the above example, preoccupation with routine care could have blinded the nurse to a possible heart attack. Technological and professional ways of being with patients also can obscure the kind of care a patient needs. Vivid presence to the patient often discloses the care needed, as Barbara Ball's care shows.

> Entering Ms. Frazier's room, I saw a frightened, angry, almost panicky woman who showed no neurological deficits other than disorientation. But she was visibly dehydrated (dry mouth, furrowed tongue, dry conjunctiva).... Her ankles and left wrist were anchored to the bed rails,

but she'd apparently broken out of the right wrist restraint, pulled out her Foley and her IV and broken the IV board at the elbow. She was tangled in bedding and wailing loudly.

Since she had apparently been "in good health" a short while ago and because she had no history of confusion, falls, or transient ischemic attacks, I decided to leave the catheter out and offer her PO fluids. Immediately, she drank 10 ounces of water and four ounces of apple juice, so I left the IV out as well.

Speaking calmly, I quieted Ms. Frazier, helped her sit up at the bedside, and changed her bedding. She didn't want to go back to bed, but I calmed her and sang her to sleep with lullabies and smooth strokes along her hands, arms, cheeks, and forehead.

During the night, I made sure Ms. Frazier was roused hourly for fluids, toileting, and neurological checks. By morning shift report, she had an intake of 1350 ml, an output of 900 ml, and was oriented and talking with anticipation about going home. She said she felt better and told us about her fall and how she'd had less than usual to drink the previous week because she'd been having a problem with urinary frequency.

Ms. Frazier was discharged home that afternoon under the watchful eye of her son and with a prescription for trimethoprim/sulfamethoxazole (Septra) and a mini-lecture on the importance of drinking enough fluids. All her neurological tests were negative.

A week later, the night-shift supervisor formally reprimanded me for not following the physician's orders, especially concerning the IV and Haldol. Apparently one of the physicians had gone straight to her to complain . . . without talking to me about the patient first.

I managed to convince the nursing supervisor that the situation did not warrant waking the intern and that my assessment of the patient had been accurate. I felt frustrated that my role as nurse was still perceived as that of handmaiden/babysitter. I was angry that anyone could be treated as Ms. Frazier had been. . . .

In Ms. Frazier's case, the supervisor and physician were focusing on acute care technologies, rather than on the unique, frightened, confused woman I saw. (Ball 1989, pp. 1466–1467)[*]

Barbara is vividly present to Ms. Frazier and her situation. Her immediate response was not to the broken wrist restraint, the pulled-out catheter, or the pulled-out IV, but to the "frightened, angry, almost panicky woman." The response of the physicians in the Emergency Department to this patient apparently had been to use the technological treatments of intravenous fluids and Foley catheter. Barbara, in contrast, had begun with vivid presence to Ms. Frazier, and from their relationship concluded that the simpler, more direct treatment of

---

[*]Reprinted from *American Journal of Nursing*, November 1989, Vol. 89, No. 11. Copyright 1989 by the American Journal of Nursing Company. Used with permission. All rights reserved.

oral fluids was indicated. In addition, her personal comforting relationship with Ms. Frazier made restraining unnecessary, understanding the patient's situation possible, and giving oral fluids an option. In short, her vivid caring presence to this unique person in a particular situation enabled her to give excellent nursing care.

Vivid presence is important in health care because, as Zaner (1981) points out, "in the bulk of our face-to-face relations, we are most often merely 'facing' one another as relative strangers, as relatively typified . . . and anonymous" (p. 232). This is often the case with nurses and patients who are assigned to each other. In the foregoing example, the nursing student became vividly present to her patient, whom she hardly knew. In addition, the nature of her vivid presence to the patient required that the patient be reflexively present to her body so that she could describe to the nurse what she experienced. In the second example, Barbara's vivid presence to an unknown patient led to appropriate care that challenged the physician's technological response and treatment.

CO-PRESENCE

Vivid presence is distinct from co-presence, according to Zaner (1981). This distinction is crucial in health care because vivid presence emphasizes reciprocal relationships between unique individuals, whereas co-presence emphasizes a mutual relationship with knowledge of the other and some degree of intimacy. Co-presence involves a mutual relationship in which both persons are present to each other as persons. In co-presence, the partners form an intimate relationship in which they "make music together" (Zaner, 1981, p. 236).

Making music together requires the partners to empower each other. Empowering each other is, for Zaner, essential to any mutual relationship. Mutual empowerment fosters freedom: "the encouraging, enabling, empowering of self to be precisely *its own self* in mutuality with the other self, which is a *potency*. That potency is . . . *freedom*" (p. 234). But giving in a mutual relationship requires "being able *to receive* the other's giving" (p. 234).

Receiving the other's giving requires awareness of the other's availability. Zaner regards availability as the essence of we-relationships. We-relationships are "experienced by each as a being-available-to one another" (p. 232). Caring relationships, obviously, require such availability. One of Zaner's most important contributions to nursing is the recognition that availability is essential to caring presence. Patients experience nurses' caring presence through their availability.

Although availability and empowerment are essential to caring presence, availability is more often associated with relationships of caring presence than is empowerment. Benner (1984) is distressed by the dissociation of empowerment from caring: "I am concerned when I hear nurses say that the very qualities essential to their caring role are the source of their powerlessness in the male-dominated hospital hierarchy" (p. 207). For her, as well as Zaner, all caring relationships require empowerment.

Zaner's co-presence, with its emphasis on empowering relationships and availability, expands our understanding of care. Caring does, as Noddings contends, involve engrossment with the experience of others and motivational shift in which we act to foster the other's well-being. But such action does require empowerment. Nurses care by acting on behalf of patients and by enabling them to care for themselves. Both types of care require nurses to be available to patients and to make that availability known. But available caring presence that fosters authentic care requires mutual empowerment that frees the patient for self-care. Combining Zaner's sense of co-presence with Noddings's sense of caring would entail a motivational shift that empowers the other to be as self-directing as possible.

The exemplar we have chosen to disclose the meaning of caring co-presence also serves as a concrete summary of the chapter. It discloses the meaning of availability, of empowerment, of engrossment, of motivational shift, of I-Thou relationships, and of triadic dialogue.

> After listening to the physician's report, I began to realize that Midori was dying. My own sadness and fear were less important than my being with her.
>
> Entering her room, I sat at the edge of Midori's bed. Her breathing was shallow and rapid. With each labored breath, her neck muscles strained and her abdomen protruded. We looked at each other, searching for the right thing to say. Only our tears came. Then silence.
>
> "Before I die, I just want to go home, pack my things, and clean up my room so my family won't have to worry about it. I just want to spend a couple of weeks with them, without their knowing that I will die soon."
>
> Her eyes focused downward as she clutched at the bed sheet. "To be honest, I would rather die while under anesthesia than suffocate to death."
>
> Then she looked at me. "I am being selfish, burdening you with all of this. I should be strong."
>
> "You are such a beautiful person," I told her. Then again we sat in silence and tears.
>
> The next morning, I was relieved to see her resting comfortably, breathing with little difficulty. During the day, she had many visitors. She had asked me earlier not to mention to anyone the seriousness of her condition. She seemed to forget the gravity of her prognosis as she unselfishly entertained her friends and family.
>
> I went in to check on her after they all left.
>
> "All my friends are so wonderful," she said. "They all care about me so much. I told them I was going home tomorrow. I didn't tell them everything."

She gathered her energy and asked me to help her wash up and take a walk. As we stood together at the mirrored basin, I saw the reflection of her small contorted body. She stood less than five feet tall—her spinal column curved to the right, an adaptation her body had made over the years, allowing her to breathe more easily. I reached for the warm, soapy washcloth and gently scrubbed her back. I could feel Midori beginning to relax as the water cleansed her body. Glancing at her reflection in the mirror, I saw a woman who suddenly looked so frail and helpless. Her body was straining, using every means to survive.

The hospital I work at is an enormous, overgrown monster—towers of steel and concrete with endless labyrinths of hallways and people scurrying in every direction. There is one place of solace, however, where a large window overlooks the city. During the day, it is like any other window, offering a view of the city's architecture, traffic, pedestrians, and an occasional helicopter. At night, however, it becomes a magical opening into the darkness where a thousand lights come alive.

I suggested to Midori that we take a walk to the window as the sun was beginning to set. Her eyes lit up when she saw the view.

"How beautiful!" she sighed.

I put my arm around her, holding her close, protecting her. I knew that this was the one place Midori could leave her illness behind.

"I just hope to go home and spend a few weeks with my family and friends."

I held her tighter.

"You know," she said, "these last two days have been the most important days of my life. I am grateful that you have helped me through them."

I left the hospital that night overwhelmed by the impact this woman had made on my life. She helped me to see nursing from a new perspective. We get all caught up in the daily routines of nursing—giving drugs, changing linens, charting. After six years in nursing, I suddenly realized what it *really* meant to be a nurse." (Dyck 1989, pp. 825).[*]

The meaning of being a nurse for Beverly is to be a caring presence to her patient. In the above case, caring presence is dialogical—that is, fully personal in the sense of Buber's I-Thou—but the dialogue is triadic in that it seeks to foster the well-being of Midori. Beverly is engrossed in her patient's situation and makes the motivational shift. She describes this shift: "My own sadness and fear were less important than my being with her." She is not only vividly co-present with her patient, but her availability invites Midori into a very intimate co-presence. Midori is empowered through caring presence in the subtle and inconspicuous ways typical of such empowerment. Her caring relationship with Beverly helps empower her to decide to live the rest of her life

---

[*]Reprinted from *American Journal of Nursing*, June 1989, Vol. 89, No. 6. Copyright 1989 by the American Journal of Nursing Company. Used with permission. All rights reserved.

with her family rather than undergo a very dangerous surgery that could take her life or leave her on a ventilator for the rest of her life. Their relationship, and especially viewing the city together, helps integrate her living and dying. Beverly's caring presence supports Midori's life-affirming way-of-being in the face of imminent death. From their relationship of caring co-presence with each other, Midori could say, "You know, these last two days have been the most important days of my life. I am grateful that you have helped me through them," and Beverly could realize "what it *really* meant to be a nurse."

STUDY QUESTIONS

1. What contributions do Anne and Jack believe caring presence can make to patient well-being? Give other examples of ways in which caring presence fosters well-being.
2. Using the example of Sarah, describe and contrast I-It and I-Thou relationships. Give examples of each relationship based on your own experience.
3. Describe an I-It(Thou) relationship. Why should nurses establish I-It(Thou) relationships with patients rather than I-It relationships?
4. Why do Anne and Jack contend that triadic dialogue is better suited for nurse-patient relationships than Buber's I-Thou dialogue?
5. Describe in your own words what Noddings means by a *caring relationship*. Give examples of caring relationships in nursing based on your own experience.
6. What implications does Noddings's distinction between natural caring and ethical caring have for nursing care? How does ethical caring address the problem of caring for those for whom nurses do not naturally care?
7. Why should natural caring be included in ethical caring?
8. Nurses often face dilemmas concerning care for patients and care for self and others. Echo Heron faced such a dilemma, as did Sheila Morgan in Case 22 in Fry & Veatch. What tensions does each face and how would you attempt to resolve them?
9. Why must limited time be considered in making moral decisions concerning nursing care?
10. Why should nursing care include empowerment? Why is it artificial to separate caring as concern from caring as practice?
11. Describe some ways that nurses can help patients be reflexively aware of their bodies.
12. Using the examples in the book, discuss the meaning of vivid presence. Why are relationships of vivid presence needed in nursing care?
13. Examine Case # 6 in Fry and Veatch in which the issue of the limits to the rights of nursing care is raised. Raise this issue in the context of the relationship of caring presence between nurse and patient. Does Mr. Williams seem vividly present to Mr. Chisholm? Do you think he could be and, if so, would it contribute to his care?

14. By interpreting Beverly's care of Midori, discuss the meaning of caring co-presence. Why are availability and empowerment necessary in relationships of co-presence?
15. Describe a "Midori presence" you have experienced. How did it affect you as a nurse and as a person?
16. In the reflexive dialogue in Chapter 7, Anne describes Beverly's care as "so subtle and unobtrusive that its quality is easily unrecognized," especially her use of silence. Give an example of when these qualities have contributed to your patient care.

REFERENCES

Ball, Barbara L. (1989). When the cure is caring. *American Journal of Nursing* 89: 1466–1467.

Benner, Patricia. (1984). *From novice to expert: Excellence and power in clinical nursing practice.* Menlo Park, CA: Addison-Wesley.

Bishop, Anne H. and John R. Scudder, Jr. (1990). *The practical, moral, and personal sense of nursing: A phenomenological philosophy of practice.* Albany, NY: State University of New York Press.

Buber, Martin. [ca. 1923] (1958). *I and thou.* 2nd ed. trans. R. G. Smith. New York: Charles Scribner's Sons.

Buber, Martin. [ca. 1923] (1970). *I and thou.* trans. W. Kaufmann. New York: Charles Scribner's Sons.

Cousins, Norman. (1989). *Head first: The biology of hope.* New York: E.P. Dutton.

Diekelmann, Nancy. (1990). Nursing education: Caring, dialogue, and practice. *Journal of Nursing Education* 29: 300–305.

Dyck, Beverly. (1989). The paper crane. *American Journal of Nursing* 89: 824–825.

Fry, S. T. and Veatch, R. M. (2000). *Case Studies in Nursing Ethics* 2nd edition. Boston, MA. Jones & Bartlett.

Gadow, Sally. (1985). Nurse and patient: The caring relationship. In A. H. Bishop and J. R. Scudder Jr. *Caring, curing, coping: Nurse, physician, patient relationships* (pp. 31–43). University, AL: University of Alabama Press.

Gilligan, Carol. (1982). *In a different voice: Psychological theory and women's development.* Cambridge, MA: Harvard University Press.

Harder, Ingegerd. (1993). *The world of the hospital nurse: Nurse patient interactions—body nursing and health promotion. Illustrated by use of a combined phenomenological/grounded theory approach.* Aarhus, Danmarks SygeplejerskehØjskole ved Aarhus Universitet, Skrift-serie fra Danmarks SygeplejerskehØjskole.

Heidegger, Martin. (1962). *Being and time.* trans. J. Macquarrie & E. Robinson. New York: Harper and Row.

Heron, Echo. (1987). *Intensive care: The story of a nurse.* New York: Ballantine.

Kohák, Erazim. (1984). *The embers and the stars: A philosophical inquiry into the moral sense of nature.* Chicago: University of Chicago Press.

Kreiger, Delores. (1981). *Foundations of holistic health nursing practices: The renaissance nurse.* Philadelphia: J. B. Lippincott.

Kwant, Ramey. C. (1965). *Phenomenology of social existence*. Pittsburgh: Duquesne University Press.

Messner, Roberta L. (1993). What patients *really* want from their nurses. *American Journal of Nursing* 93(8): 38–41.

Moyers, Bill. (1989). *A world of ideas*. New York: Doubleday.

Noddings, Nel. (1984). *Caring: A feminine approach to ethics and moral education*. Berkeley: University of California Press.

Nussbaum, Martha C. (1986). *The fragility of goodness: Luck and ethics in Greek tragedy and philosophy*. Cambridge: Cambridge University Press.

Quinn, Janet. (1981). Client care and nurse involvement in a holistic framework. In D. Kreiger (Ed.), *Foundations of holistic health nursing practices: The renaissance nurse* (pp. 197–210). Philadelphia: J. B. Lippincott.

Scudder, John R. Jr. (1990). Dependent and authentic care: Implications of Heidegger for nursing care. In M. Leininger and J. Watson (Eds.), *The caring imperative in education*, (pp. 59–75). New York: National League for Nursing.

Scudder, John R. Jr., and Algis Mickunas. (1985). *Meaning, dialogue, and enculturation: Phenomenological philosophy of education*. Washington, DC: Center for Advanced Research in Phenomenology: University Press of America.

Zaner, Richard M. (1981). *The context of self: A phenomenological inquiry using medicine as a clue*. Athens, OH: Ohio University Press.

Zaner, Richard M. (1985). "How the hell did I get here?" Reflections on being a patient. In Anne H. Bishop and John R. Scudder, Jr. (Eds.), *Caring, curing, coping: Nurse, physician, patient relationships* (p. 80–105). University, AL.: University of Alabama Press.

Zaner, Richard M. (1993). *Troubled voices: Stories of ethics and illness*. Cleveland, OH: Pilgrim Press.

Chapter

Called to Care

Nurses like Beverly and patients like Midori call us to care. Beverly calls us to be caring persons through her example of caring; Midori calls us to care through her need for care, and her authentic, sensitive way of eliciting care. In Noddings's terms, Midori calls us through natural care and Beverly through ethical care. Encountering a patient like Midori evokes natural caring. Encountering a caring person like Beverly evokes a desire to be such a person.

Evocative examples that call us to care foster integral care. Integral care is a way-of-being with others in which the desire to care, the purpose of care, the meaning of care, and the act of caring are one. In our time, we have dismembered integral care by assigning the desire to care to psychology, the meaning of caring to philosophy, and the practice of caring to those concerned with procedures and methodology. This separation is assumed when exemplars of moral excellence are used to arouse feelings rather than to evoke a way-of-being. So-called charismatic speakers—some promoters, politicians, and preachers—make it their goal to manipulate the feelings of others. Listeners often respond to these speakers by feeling ennobled rather than acting nobly. In contrast, when meaning, feelings, and actions are not separated, examples of caring call persons into caring ways-of-being.

Being Called to Care

Peggy Chinn (1994) contends that being called to care is an appropriate description of evoking that way-of-being called *integral care*.

> "Calling" can mean the power of naming. "A call" can mean the power of purpose. "Being called" can mean the existence that is signified by naming, as well as the fuel for action that is fired by purpose. "Called

to care" is a willingness to Be in significant relation, to be responsive to others, to be in spirit together, in human existence together. In a deeply spiritual sense, it is the highest calling. In a profoundly practical sense, it is the most urgent calling beckoning all people on the earth today. (Chinn, 1994, vii)

Chinn contends that interpreting care as a potential way of being into which we are called is an appropriate way of understanding caring.

The human potential to care, like the human potential to be authentic, cannot be classified or characterized as a single "thing," nor can it conform to classifications. It cannot be boxed, packaged, or delivered on command. As a human potential, it can be envisioned, it can be imagined, it can be experienced, it can be learned, it can be nurtured. Caring can be called forth; it can be inspired. It can be called forth from any human. As a potential, it can be developed more fully as it is practiced, understood, responded to, explored, envisioned. (Chinn, 1994, viii)

Caring is called forth by envisioning future possibilities for well-being. A possible future project that seems destined to foster human well-being calls us into action. In contrast to the future orientation of calling, some ethical considerations involve using a universal ethical principle to make rational judgments about moral choices that prescribe moral actions. The principle used is believed to have religious or philosophical foundations that are good for all times. Those who challenge this approach often point out the difficulty in establishing that one principle is preferable to others: for instance, in health care, the principle of autonomy or the principle of the greatest good for the greatest number. Interpreting ethics as a call to care challenges this approach by contending that the good is brought about by focusing on possibilities for fostering human well-being in the future. Thus, rather than seeking moral imperatives that require conformity based on a fixed system, moral imperative comes as an invitation to foster good by realizing future possibilities. The call to care comes as an invitation to share in a relationship that will foster future human well-being.

Nurses usually experience the call to care in everyday practice as particular visions that promise to foster the well-being of their patients. They seldom think of these visions as calls to care, but merely as sound nursing care. The good to be fostered by nursing practice is so inherent in nursing care that it usually is not explicitly apparent to the care giver. The call to care present in nursing practice often is explicitly recognized when unusual circumstances bring it to light. One aforementioned nurse recognized her calling when a mother profusely thanked her for saving her baby's life by giving mouth-to-mouth resuscitation. Although the nurse responded by saying that any competent nurse could and would have given mouth-to-mouth, her decision to remain in nursing indicates that she heard and responded to the call to care inherent in nursing practice.

The call to care is so inherent in nursing practice that nurses who enter nursing with no sense of call to care often find it in their practice.

> I'll have to confess that I never did feel called into nursing. I feel like I fell into nursing. I think it had a lot to do with life experiences and situations, social contexts that I was embedded in at the time. I had the opportunity to have some work experiences in a hospital setting that oriented me to nursing. I had choices to make in college. I really didn't know what I wanted to do with my life. That was something I was familiar with. It was more comfortable and less threatening to enter into. As I learned more about nursing, as I got into the profession, I grew into it. I grew to love it, but I definitely did not feel called from the very beginning. (Lashley, Neal, Slunt, Berman, & Hultgren, 1994, p. 7)

The preceding "confession" is given by Mary Lashley, one of the authors of *Being Called to Care*. The call to care obviously did not initiate her entry into nursing, but became her calling through engaging in nursing practice with its inherent moral sense of care. Her call came from participating in nursing practice that presupposes being called to care.

THE "OF COURSE" RESPONSE TO CALLS TO CARE

The nurse who gave mouth-to-mouth resuscitation was ready to leave nursing when the child's mother called her back into nursing by praising her. The nurse responded by saying, in effect, "Of course, I gave mouth-to-mouth. Any nurse would respond as I did." Most calls to care in nursing occur in this way. The nurse is also saying, in effect, "What I did is no big deal." Many ethicists want to reserve ethical designation only for "big deals." They contend that care given out of a desire to foster well-being of a particular person in a situation is not ethical care. For example, Noddings contends that care can be called ethical when it is done out of the desire to be a caring person or out of valuing caring as such, but not when it is done out of spontaneous natural concern.

The nurse who gave the infant mouth-to-mouth assumed that any nurse would desire to keep a child from dying and would have the requisite skill to do it. Beverly's care for Midori was no "big deal" in this sense. She desired to comfort and support Midori and had the interpersonal skills needed to do it. Her interpersonal skills are both those required of nurses and those of sensitive human beings. Her helping Midori arrive at the decision for no treatment is a nursing skill. Her taking Midori to see a beautiful sight is the care of a sensitive person. In neither case is there any evidence of her acting out of duty, out of the desire to be a caring nurse, or out of valuing caring as such. She cares for Midori spontaneously and naturally in a way that discloses the integral relationship of the sentiment of care and the practice of care and the integral relationship between being a good nurse and being a good person.

Pellegrino: The Call of Profession

Edmund Pellegrino (1985) shows the integral relationship between the sentiment of care and the practice of care and between being a good physician or nurse and being a good person by disclosing the moral sense of a profession. He contends that the word *profession* originally referred to "a special promise to help humanity and to place it above one's own interest. This has always been the doctor's special promise, his common devotion, and the source of his ethical obligations" (1985, p. 28). To the degree that physicians and nurses accept Pellegrino's moral sense of profession, they will respond to their patient's plight with "of course." His stress on the moral nature of profession speaks forcefully to nurses as well as physicians, although he illustrates this moral sense with examples taken from the physician-patient relationship. He contends that the physician-patient relationship begins with a concrete request for care made by a person who is ill and seeks help. The physician accepts this request for help by the act of profession, in which the physician professes to be able to help the patient and to use her/his ability for the patient's well-being. This promise to use knowledge and skill for the well-being of the patient is, for Pellegrino, the essence of a profession. Thus, a profession has a moral foundation in which the professional professes to foster the well-being of those seeking help. For Pellegrino, health care professionals engage in health care by affirmative response to the call to care.

Pellegrino (1985) believes that both nursing and medicine share a common imperative to care for the ill and debilitated. There are four ways of caring in Pellegrino's interpretation of integral care. The first is compassion; the second is doing for others what they cannot do for themselves because of illness and debilitation; the third is using knowledge and skill to care for the patient; the fourth is care involving the craft of health care (Pellegrino, 1985). Regardless of differences in nursing and medical care, a caring relationship does call both nurse and physician into relationships with patients that involve compassion, direct care, knowledge and skill, and craft.

Sara Fry (1989) disagrees with Pellegrino's contention that an interpretation of caring developed for a physician-patient relationship is adequate for nurse-patient relationships. Even though we believe that Pellegrino's description of caring relationships in health care makes important contributions to nursing, we agree with Fry that his approach seems more appropriate for physician-patient than for nurse-patient relationships. His description of caring assumes that the health care giver and the patient choose each other. In most nursing situations, this is rarely true for nurse or patient. In addition, although Pellegrino points this out, physicians rarely do for patients what they cannot do for themselves, such as bathing. Nurses, too, are less involved in such activities than they once were, although many recognize that personal care such as bathing affords an excellent opportunity for developing the nurse-patient relationship. Nevertheless, basic nursing care often requires more intimate relationships between nurse and patient than the relationship between physician and patient. In addition, Pellegrino focuses moral decision making on securing agreement between what is *medically* indicated and what is called for by the patient's view of the good life. What is medically indicated usually means prescribing a particular treatment, whereas nursing involves continuous, ongoing care. Nurses often hear patients say, "It hurts to move," "I don't want to eat this food," "Don't make me get up," when restoring good health requires a patient to do all of these. Rather than prescribing, nurses engage in persuasive interaction that responds to patient desires. Nursing care usually concerns ongoing care in which there is interaction between nurse and patient that calls for continual informing consent between what good nursing care requires and what the patient desires.

Regardless of differences between nursing care and medical care, Pellegrino eliminates the bifurcation between professional care and moral care that plagues both medicine and nursing. For him, although professionals require special knowledge and skills, the essential meaning of professional is to be called to care.

JAMES: CONCRETE CALLING

William James (1948), like Pellegrino, believed that we are called to be moral by our interaction with persons. James contends that we are called to moral action when others make concrete demands on us. He maintained "that without a claim actually made by some concrete person there can be no obligation, but that there is some obligation wherever there is a claim" (James, 1948, p. 72). Thus for James, as for Pellegrino, the call to care is given concretely by specific persons.

The concrete call to care, for James, comes not only from specific persons but from the situations to which persons respond. He was wary of the idealistic version of calls to morality that were divorced from specific situations. He described such utopian divorcement from the world during a visit to a Chautauqua retreat. His feelings were elevated by the pleasant surroundings, wonderful lectures, good conversations, and excellent concerts. He described it as a middle-class heaven. Eventually he became uneasy because he felt divorced from the struggle and tension always present in the "real world."

As he journeyed from Lake Chautauqua, he passed through the steel mills of Buffalo and saw the laborers sweating and straining under conditions typical of most factory work in the latter nineteenth century in America. He then recalled how Tolstoy and others idealized the work of the common laborer. But when he examined the life of the common worker who merely struggled to exist, he found it wanting.

> The barrenness and ignobleness of the more usual laborer's life consist in the fact that it is moved by no such ideal inner springs. The backache, the long hours, the danger, are patiently endured—for what? To

gain a quid of tobacco, a glass of beer, a cup of coffee, a meal, and a bed, and to begin again the next day and shirk as much as one can. (James, 1958, p. 185)

Then he concluded that hard work and struggle alone did not make life worth living.

A life was worth living, for James, when moral vision of possible good called a person into a new way-of-being. This vision was not a general one addressed to everyone, but a concrete one. In living in specific situations with specific talents, a person would be called by a vision of possible good specifically addressed to the particular person at a certain time.

James's approach to ethics is evident in the relationship of Beverly and Midori. Midori's plight called Beverly into a caring relationship with her. The quality of that relationship gave Beverly a new vision of what it meant to be a good nurse, a vision that promised to inspire and guide her future nursing care. This interpretation of concrete calling is well suited to nursing ethics. Nurses are in situations in which the plight of the ill, the injustice of the situation, and the nature of their talents all call them to care in specific ways. James's contention that responding to moral calling makes life worth living is supported by our study of fulfillment in nursing (Bishop & Scudder, 1990). In that study, 39 of 40 nurses described their most fulfilling experiences as a nurse as ones in which they fulfilled their moral calling in specific situations.

JESUS: CALLED BY THE PLIGHT OF THE NEIGHBOR

A classic example of nursing care given out of the desire to help a particular person in a concrete situation is the story of the Good Samaritan. The goal of the story is not disclosing the meaning of nursing care but that of being a neighbor. Jesus tells the story not only to disclose the meaning of being a neighbor, but also to evoke compassion for those in need and to issue a call to care for them. He rejects a lawyer's request for an academic definition of *neighbor* and gives a concrete one in a parable.

> [30]"... A man was going down from Jerusalem to Jericho, and fell among robbers, who stripped him and beat him, and departed, leaving him half dead. [31]Now by chance a priest was going down that road; and when he saw him he passed by on the other side. [32]So likewise a Levite, when he came to the place and saw him, passed by on the other side. [33]But a Samaritan, as he journeyed, came to where he was; and when he saw him, he had compassion, [34]and went to him and bound up his wounds, pouring on oil and wine; then he set him on his own beast and brought him to an inn, and took care of him. [35]And the next day he took out two denarii and gave them to the innkeeper, saying, 'Take care

of him; and whatever more you spend, I will repay you when I come back.' ³⁶Which of these three, do you think, proved neighbor to the man who fell among the robbers?" ³⁷He said, "The one who showed mercy on him." And Jesus said to him, "Go and do likewise." (Luke 10:30–37)

From the point of view of traditional philosophy, the dialogue between Jesus and the lawyer in verses 36 and 37 is disappointing. A philosopher would expect Jesus to give a definition of *neighbor* after giving such an excellent example of the meaning of *neighbor*. Instead, Jesus's question "Which of these three do you think proved neighbor to the man who fell among the robbers?" subtly questions the intent of the lawyer. By his question, Jesus redirects the concern of the lawyer from an academic definition of neighbor to the concrete relationship of being a good neighbor. His concluding imperative, "Go and do likewise," indicates that knowing the meaning of being a neighbor issues a call to neighborly care.

The neighborly care exemplified by the Good Samaritan is nursing care. The Samaritan responds to the injured person by pouring oil and wine on the wounds, bandaging them, by caring for the victim for the remainder of the day, and by arranging for his recuperative care. But his call is to the nursing care of the common life. He is not a professional nurse specifically dedicated to caring for the injured with the specialized skill and knowledge that empowers that care.

Does being empowered as a nurse imply being available for care outside of health care institutions? The priest and Levite obviously did not believe that their special priestly abilities for care should be used with persons who were not part of their professional responsibilities. In contrast, the Samaritan felt called to care for a person who was probably a Jew, not a Samaritan. We do not know the injured man's religious tradition because the Samaritan responded to him as a person who needed care, and not as someone for whom he had specific responsibility.

Having a similar sense of calling, a nurse responded to the call to care for three elderly neighbors when they were ill. She responded as a neighbor, but as a specially empowered neighbor when health care was needed. Her response to their needs and their calling on her was predicated on her nursing ability and skill. She believed that nurses are called to care, not by their institutional employment, but by concern for the well-being of persons and by having a special empowerment to foster their well-being. The Good Samaritan is different from this nurse only in lacking special empowerment to engage in nursing care. Although this nurse had much greater proficiency in nursing care than the Samaritan, she was called to care by the plight of those who needed care in the same way that the Samaritan was called.

WERNER MARX: CALLED BY COMPASSION

Werner Marx (1992) develops an ethics of compassion that is not founded in the Judeo-Christian tradition. He asserts that his search for another foundation for an ethics of compassion is not based on opposition to the Judeo-Christian tradition. He simply recognizes that this foundation is no longer available to many persons (Marx, p. 43). His attempt to develop such an ethics discloses his belief that the best ethics is one of compassion.

He attempts to found his ethics of compassion on the shared mortality of all humans. He believes that when we honestly face our mortality, "horror . . ., in the true sense of the word" shatters the comfortable, everyday world in which we dwell (Marx, 1992, pp. 48–49). When I dwell securely within this taken-for-granted way-of-being, I tend to be indifferent to others and to my own mortality. When the horror of my mortality shatters this indifference, I am open to the presence of others as fellow human beings. Isolated and forlorn, I need the presence of my brother or sister. Then, "I am not only able to *see* the other as my other . . . but also to *hear* his *call*" (p. 52).

When I see and hear my neighbors, I recognize them as sharing my fate. But does this shared fate make them my neighbors? For Marx, it does not necessarily make them neighbors, but does free me from the "captivity of indifference" that prevents them from being my neighbors. When I am freed from indifference, I am freed to respond to the other's call to brotherhood or sisterhood. Responding to the other's call means that I treat her/him as an equal and with compassion.

Nurses care for patients who are being forced to face their own mortality in ways that can open them to the need for compassionate relations with others. Nurses often respond to patients by relating to them in the conventional ways of the profession. They are often shocked out of treating this person as *the* patient in *this* professionally defined way by confronting their own mortality through their patient's mortality. Mutual facing of mortality often calls nurse and patient out of their shell of conventionality into authentic, compassionate care for each other.

Facing mortality opens up the possibility of personal relationships, according to Marx, because people reach out for personal, compassionate relationships. He believes that a person is always searching out others saying, "Notice me, acknowledge me, relieve me from my loneliness, have compassion for me, love me" (p. 60). When responded to with love and compassion, a person rejoices: "The fulfillment of the call of the person waiting for neighborly love releases joy in him, joy at having been heard, at having been listened to. . . . Joy 'is infectious'. . . . Joy . . . makes 'brothers' of all men wherever it dwells" (p. 60).

For Marx, being with others as brothers and sisters makes life worth living and fills it with joy. The purpose of facing our mortality is to shatter the habitual indifference that inhibits reaching out for brotherhood/sisterhood and compassion. Marx's emphasis on the shock of facing our own mortality, however, seems to keep him from recognizing that his ethics of compassion is rooted in the human desire for compassion and brotherhood/sisterhood rather than in our common mortality.

A nurse who took part in our study of fulfillment in nursing describes how compassionate caring for a dying patient brought her joy and her greatest fulfillment as a nurse.

> Two years ago I had the opportunity to deliver total patient care to a 25-year-old girl with end stage congestive cardiomyopathy. She was in congestive heart failure with many ventricular life threatening arrhythmias. She was well aware of the fact that she was going to die and admitted her fright to me and also asked me point blank if she was going to die. We were able to discuss such problems as how could this be explained to her 7-year-old daughter? Who would care for her 7-year-old daughter and her own 16-year-old retarded sister? I also discussed with her family, some of the fears she acknowledged and encouraged them to discuss these things with her. Her main request of me was that I sit by her during the night and simply hold her hand. In addition to ministering to these needs, I also monitored her vital signs, changes in physical assessment, titrating various vasopressors and vasodilators to maintain optimum cardiac output. I overrode our strict visiting policies to allow her husband and daughter to sit at her bedside as they wished with the understanding that they would promptly leave if asked to do so by any of us. This patient remained in my unit for 4–5 weeks in critical condition before dying, and though we all felt the hurt of losing her, we also felt the joy obtained by providing emotional and physical support along with patient teaching to both patient and family and helped both patient and family to accept and begin to deal with her inevitable death. (Scudder & Bishop, 1990, pp. 95–96)

The preceding example illustrates how facing death calls patient and nurse into an intimate relationship that supports and comforts the dying person and brings joy in the face of tragedy. An even more poignant example of how personal relationships can help persons face death will be evident in the example of the care of Lara in the next chapter.

Taylor: The Call to Authenticity

Whereas Marx develops an ethics of compassion that issues a call to care, Charles Taylor (1991) gives a philosophical interpretation of the ethics of authenticity that can call nurses to care. The call to care implicit in an ethics of authenticity is often missed because, as Taylor points out, neither the critics nor the defenders of authenticity do justice to its ethical import. The defenders and critics both place authenticity within an ethical relativism that makes choice itself focal. Taylor points out that choice is insignificant without some means of determining that one choice is better than another. He contends that authenticity is morally significant when it commits persons to choose to pursue the best, given their potential and situation in the world.

> The moral ideal behind self-fulfillment is that of being true to oneself, in a specifically modern understanding of that term. . . . What do I mean by moral ideal? I mean a picture of what a better or higher mode

of life would be, where "better" and "higher" are defined not in terms of what we happen to desire or need, but offer a standard of what we ought to desire. (Taylor, 1991, pp. 15–16).

This interpretation of authenticity can enlighten Noddings's ethical caring. In her interpretation of caring, when I do not care naturally, I should care because I want to be a caring person. Translated into nursing, this would mean that I care for clients even when I do not naturally care for them because I recognize caring as the way I ought to be. In so doing, I would be authentic in that I would be following the vision of what I "ought to desire," namely being in a caring relationship that fosters the well-being of others. Thus, a nurse who cares for patients because she/he wants to become a caring person would be an authentic nurse, just as would be a nurse who cared out of natural caring, because both are being led by what they ought to desire: being in a caring relationship that fosters the well-being of their patients.

Taylor's interpretation of the moral sense of authenticity is valuable to nurses who wish to foster authenticity in patients by giving them authentic care. We have previously discussed authentic care in the following way.

> Heidegger (1962) . . . contrasts two ways of caring for others. In the first way, a person will *"leap in"* for another and "take over for the other." This form of care can readily foster domination and dependency when the caregiver "leaps in and takes away 'care.' " We will call this dependent care because it fosters dependency on others. In contrast to dependent care, authentic care (so named by Heidegger) occurs when the care giver will *"leap ahead* of him [ihm vorausspringt] in his existentiell (sic) potentiality-for-Being, not in order to take away his 'care' but rather to give it back to him authentically" (pp. 158–159). Thus, in authentic care the other is helped to care for his or her own being. (Bishop & Scudder, 1991, p. 56)

Nurses who have been in practice for a long time will recognize that much of the care given earlier in this century was dependent care. Increasingly nurses have become aware of the value of authentic care that frees patients to direct their own being. Such care requires greater emphasis on patient education and encouraging clients to take responsibility for their health care, as Dorothea Orem (1985) advocated. Taylor's moral sense of authenticity would require nurses to move a step further by helping persons to discover possibilities for becoming their best selves during and after illness and treatment.

Sally Gadow's (1980) contention that nurses ought to be existential advocates calls for nurses to help patients become more authentic by the way they care for them. By *existential advocacy,* she means helping patients discover the meaning of illness and treatment for their lives and encouraging and assisting them in following that meaning. The nurse as existential advocate does not merely help patients choose what they want—for example, the drug user who wants to be as "high" as possible while in the hospital. The existential advocate is there to help patients recognize and realize their best selves, given their situation.

The stress in medical ethics on decisions concerning treatment or nontreatment often obscures the moral imperative to assist patients in discovering and pursuing their best selves in a given health care situation. This is evident in the case that we discussed in the first chapter in which a patient with mania refused to take Lithium because he wanted to remain high. Both the ethicist and the physicians were so focused on the issue of whether to treat or not to treat that they failed to discuss with the patient the moral issues involved in his decision not to take Lithium. They seemed not to recognize the moral imperative to help the patient discover and realize his best self. Ethical considerations could have led this patient to consider what would be best for his life rather than merely what would foster his pleasure. Such considerations make ethics an integral aspect of health care because they involve helping patients discover and choose what they ought to desire for future well-being rather than what they presently desire. For example, an elderly person with a broken hip desires to avoid pain, but her nurse encourages her to face the pain in order to be able to walk again and thus become a more independent person.

That moral considerations could be an essential ingredient in practice itself is often obscured by the tendency to interpret nursing as an applied or behavioral science. This interpretation often denies that persons are capable of desiring and choosing to pursue future possible good in given situations—an assumption that underlies Taylor's interpretation of authenticity. Social scientists do this, according to Taylor, by attributing behavior to non-moral factors such as the desire for survival, power, control, or wealth in an attempt to give explanations that are "hard" and "scientific" (Taylor, 1991, p. 20). Applying this stance in nursing, as we have argued in our previous books, has blinded nurses to the moral sense inherent in its practice. Consequently, we believe, with Taylor, that retrieval of "this ideal can help us restore our practice" (p. 23).

An ethics of authenticity makes its claim on me in a way uniquely appropriate to my way-of-being and my situation, according to Taylor. This unique calling means that my identity cannot be "socially derived but must be inwardly generated" (p. 47). Forming my identity requires inward generation called forth by the world.

> I alone experience myself as a subject, but I experience myself in a world that makes demands on me and in interaction with others that fosters self-understanding. Inward generation of self-definition is initiated by a call from the world. . . . Only if I exist in a world in which history, or the demands of nature, or the needs of my fellow human beings, or the duties of citizenship, or the call of God, or something else of this order *matters* crucially, can I define an identity for myself that is not trivial. Authenticity is not the enemy of demands that emanate from beyond the self; it supposes such demands. (Taylor, 1991, pp. 40–41)

The call to moral commitment that emanates from beyond the self is often given by working with others through "horizons of significance" (Taylor, p. 38). In nursing, these horizons of significance constitute the meanings that orient nursing practice. A nurse does not define herself/himself out of an inward generation divorced from practice, but through the meanings embedded in practice. The essential meaning of practice is a moral sense: caring for the well-being of others.

Novice nurses who have a strong sense of being called to care often have difficulty relating this call to the practice of nursing. We found in our study of fulfillment in nursing that nursing students need to learn how the call to care is carried out in practice. The 40 senior nursing students we compared with 40 practicing nurses felt most fulfilled when care referred to personal relationships. But these relationships, unlike those of the experienced nurses, tended to be divorced from the practice of caring for patients in clinical situations. For example, one nursing student, who regarded nursing as "being enabled to care empathetically for those less fortunate," described her most fulfilling nursing experience as being at the beck and call of her patient to do favors that had marginal relationship to nursing practice. In contrast, in the descriptions of care for patients by experienced nurses, the personal and moral were so often disclosed in professional and technical language that Jack often needed a translation into lay terms by Anne in order for him to grasp the moral and personal significance of their care. Regardless of how technical the descriptions of the care that brought these nurses fulfillment, they were all examples of fulfilling the moral sense of nursing in ways that were responses to the call to care given in actual practice (Bishop & Scudder, 1990).

If our study accurately depicts the prevalence of the moral sense in nursing, why are the moral sense and the call to care so neglected? Nurses are socialized to describe their nursing experiences in the technical and professional language of nursing in ways that obscure the moral sense and the sense of being called to care. In nursing literature and education, the term *professional* is often substituted for the moral imperative. When nurses do not practice as they ought to practice, they usually are not charged with being "immoral," but with being "unprofessional." For example, when nurses abandon a patient needing constant supervision in order to gossip with colleagues in the lounge, they are usually charged with being unprofessional rather than immoral. The charge of immorality is usually reserved for cases that are included under such terms as *moral turpitude*. Charges of moral turpitude are usually concerned with unacceptable conduct that seldom directly affects patient care.

Nurses are charged with being unprofessional when they deviate from professionally established criteria. This way of thinking comes from interpreting nursing as a profession in the sociological rather than the moral sense. The sociological definition of profession includes having a body of knowledge, educational standards, criteria for judging competent performance, and a code of ethics. One motivating factor in developing the code of ethics for nursing has been to establish nursing as a profession. This probably accounts for the failure of the code to give significant direction to nursing practice, even when the code sets sound standards for what nursing ought to be.

One problem with the sociological definition of profession is that it is arrived at by consensus. Definition by consensus eliminates the moral sense. Morality cannot be determined by consensus without losing the normative sense that is essential to morality. Pellegrino (1985) makes this clear in his moral interpretation of profession. He argues that the American Medical Association (AMA) puts the cart before the horse in contending that the AMA Code of Ethics is morally binding because it has been proclaimed by the leadership of the AMA as the consensus of the medical profession. For Pellegrino, medicine is a profession if, and only if, it is true to what it professes: namely, to use medical skill and knowledge to foster the well-being of the patient. A profession receives its special privileges from living up to its moral profession. Therefore, the profession does not establish the moral sense. The moral sense constitutes the profession.

Another way in which the moral sense of nursing is obscured is by viewing nursing as a morally neutral technological activity. Technology, for Taylor, is a concrete form of the instrumental reason that has become the dominant way of thinking in our society. He points out that both critics of instrumental reasoning and its uncritical advocates usually put it in a framework of dominance and control. Unfortunately, neither critics nor advocates seek a context for technology other than domination.

The uncritical advocates of instrumental reason, according to Taylor, believe that it is *the* way to solve all of our problems. They situate problems so that the technical sense, rather than moral sense, has priority by neglecting that which is specifically human.

> We are embodied agents, living in dialogical conditions, inhabiting time in a specifically human way, that is, making sense of our life as a story that connects the past from which we have come to our future projects. That means . . . that if we are properly to treat a human being, we have to respect this embodied, dialogical, temporal nature. (Taylor, 1991, pp. 105–106)

Taylor points out that the neglect of the human and the moral often takes place in medicine.

> Runaway extensions of instrumental reason, such as the medical practice that forgets the patient as a person, that takes no account of how the treatment relates to his or her story and thus of the determinants of hope and despair, that neglects the essential rapport between caregiver and patient—all these have to be resisted in the name of the moral background in benevolence that justifies these applications of instrumental reason themselves. If we come to understand why technology is important here in the first place, then it will of itself be limited and enframed by an ethic of caring. (Taylor, 1991, p. 106)

Nurses who place technology in the context of dominance can learn much from Taylor's critique of instrumental reasoning. Advocates of technology who place it in the context of dominating nature usually regard nursing primarily as intervention. Nurses who favor a humanistic approach to nursing often grudgingly admit that technology can contribute to nursing care. Unfortunately, they often limit ethics to personal relations in nursing, neglecting technology. Those nurses who fail to engage in moral critique of instrumental reason often fall into ways of speaking and thinking that help transform nursing into a technology. This is especially true when nurses uncritically adopt the language of intervention. In so doing, they call everything they do for or with patients "interventions," even when such language makes no sense. For example, one nursing scholar lists as interventions to treat hopelessness: "compliment on appearances and/or efforts when appropriate," and "encourage verbalization to determine the client's perception of choices" (Carpenito, 1995, p. 488). Obviously, the preceding are not interventions but moral responses of human beings to other human beings who are facing a common human condition. Hopelessness is loss of prospects for future well-being, not a disease that requires intervention. Nurses can assist those who have lost hope by helping them see possibilities for future well-being and supporting them in realizing their possibilities (Bishop & Scudder, 1991, pp. 43–49).

Taylor shows that technology belongs in a context other than dominance. He contends that we need to understand technology "in the moral frame of the ethic of practical benevolence" (Taylor, 1991, p. 106). This is especially needed for nurses who practice in highly technical situations. They are no less called to care than those whose practice involves more hands-on and personal care. They are called to care technically. But if the call to technical efficiency is their primary calling, they are technicians rather than nurses. This does not mean that technical efficiency is unimportant or that nurses should not feel pride and fulfillment from technical competency. It does mean that a nurse's call to be technical must be enframed in an ethics of care. The ultimate call for nurses is the call to care. The call to care, unlike the contingent call of technical competence, is itself a moral calling, as is evident in the following example.

> One nurse described a patient who had undergone an aneurysm clipping, as a "GCS5T, E4, M1, VT [who] opened his eyes but [had] no movement and was trached.... I can't describe the sensation I felt; but to see him follow a command for the first time—moving his thumb—made me feel wonderful inside. All of our diligent nursing care, positioning, ROM, stimulation, etc. was working and it felt good." Interestingly, in a follow-up interview with this nurse, she stated that although this work was very technical, she would not remain in nursing if it were not for personal and moral fulfillment. (Bishop and Scudder, 1990, pp. 99–100)

This nurse has obviously succeeded in enframing highly technical nursing care in "an ethic of technical benevolence" (Taylor, 1991, p. 106).

Taylor's treatment of technology discloses the method he uses throughout his book, *The Ethics of Authenticity* (1991). He attempts to "identify and articulate the higher ideal behind . . . practices, and then criticize these practices from the standpoint of their own motivating ideal" (p. 72). Instead of dismissing or endorsing a practice, Taylor contends that we ought to make evident what it means in terms of its motivating ideal and then point out what being true to that ideal really involves. Taylor's method, when applied to the purpose of this book, would require us to identify the essential and authentic meaning of nursing practice and then to test and judge the worth of nursing practice by the extent to which it fulfills its moral sense. We have, without explicitly following Taylor's approach, used a similar approach in our attempt to develop a nursing ethic. We have claimed that nursing is the practice of caring and that it has the inherent moral sense of fostering the well-being of others. This means that nursing ethics would primarily concern how well the moral sense of nursing is being fulfilled by individual nurses and by the nursing profession. In addition, since the worth of nursing itself would be judged by how it fulfills its moral sense, moral concerns would not be peripheral or add-on concerns to nursing's professional and technical activities, but would form the very heart of nursing practice itself.

THE INTEGRAL CALLING OF COMPASSION AND AUTHENTICITY

If moral calling is to act out of compassion to care for the well-being of clients, can nurses be expected to respond authentically to this calling? It would make no sense to say that nurses ought to be compassionate in the same way that we say nurses should act to foster the well-being of patients. Being compassionate is not something that human beings can achieve by an act of will. It is possible, however, to be open to compassion, to be situated so that compassion is likely to be evoked, and to follow the call of compassion.

In the parable of the Good Samaritan, the priest and the Levite who passed by on the other side, in contrast to the Samaritan, were not open to the calling and direction of compassion. The ethical question with regard to compassion should not be "Ought I be compassionate?" but rather "Ought I be open to compassion, to give myself to it, and to act out of it?" Acting compassionately usually finds itself in tension with other ways-of-being, such as self-serving, detached objective observation, seeking the truth, comfort-seeking, cowardly retreat, or desiring the approval of others. Thus, an ethics of compassion concerns being open to the call of compassion and being willing to respond to that call by fostering the well-being of the person whose situation initially evoked the compassion. The Good Samaritan is morally commendable not because he felt compassion, but because he was open to compassion and allowed it to foster good nursing care for the injured person. The Good Samaritan is authentic in that his nursing care follows naturally from his compassion, and he chose to act out of that compassion.

What of nurses who do not feel compassion but feel called to care? They can, according to Noddings, be called to care out of the desire to be a caring person by entering a caring relationship with those who need care. I am moral when I choose to be in that caring way that fosters the well-being of others. This, according to Taylor, would make me authentic, in that I am choosing to follow what I ought to desire—being in caring relationships with those who need my care. Thus, I can be an authentic person by choosing to follow compassion or by choosing what I ought to desire: to be a caring person. In nursing when I choose to authentically follow compassion, I naturally foster the well-being of my clients. When compassion is not present, I am called to care by my desire to be a caring nurse and by the caring way-of-being evoked by nursing practice.

Choosing to be a caring nurse requires me to engage in a caring relationship focused on fostering the patient's well-being. The moral sense of nursing practice invites me to enter authentically into caring relationships with my clients and gives me ways of caring for their well-being. In authentic care, we are called to care out of a desire to be caring persons and to be excellent practitioners who care for the well-being of clients. In compassionate care, we are called directly to care for their well-being. When the call to care is a call to act out of compassion, out of the desire to be a caring nurse, and out of authentic participation in caring practice, three powerful sources of morality come together to foster compassionate, authentic care for those whose plight calls for care.

STUDY QUESTIONS

1. In what ways does the relationship of Beverly and Midori call nurses to care? What are some other ways?
2. Why does Chinn believe that being called to care is the appropriate way to speak of becoming a caring person?
3. Some critics of contemporary morality argue that the only way to restore the moral fiber of our people is to return to the philosophical and religious foundations that once called people to care. Others argue that such contentions merely state the problem rather than offering the solution to our lack of moral conviction. The problem is that we no longer accept and respond to traditional moral foundations. With which position do you agree? Why?
4. What do Jack and Anne mean by the "of course" response to calls to care? Do you think that most moral acts in nursing occur as "of course" responses? Why or why not?
5. Why does Pellegrino say that the AMA has the cart before the horse when it contends that the AMA's Code of Ethics is valid because it speaks for the majority of physicians? How does Pellegrino believe that ethics and professions are related to each other? What implication does his interpretation of profession have for nursing?

6. What are the four ways of caring in Pellegrino's interpretation of integral care? Do you agree with Fry's contention that Pellegrino's caring relationship is inadequate for nursing? Why or why not?
7. What are the implications of James's "concrete calling" for nursing care? Give an example of a concrete call to care that you have experienced. In Case #53 in Fry & Veatch, in which doing good may harm the patient, the good that Joan Schuller is called to support is a patient's violating of hospital procedures in order to give her child the best neonatal experience. Can you think of examples of being called to care by confronting unexpected situations?
8. How is the call to care given to the Good Samaritan different from that of a nurse? How is it similar?
9. Why does Marx contend that facing our mortality opens us to the possibility of compassionate and neighborly relationships with others? What implications does his contention have for nurses who are helping patients face death?
10. Why does Taylor reject choosing what we want or need as the meaning of authenticity? Why does he reject placing authenticity in a context of dominance? Give examples of claims to being authentic in nursing that Taylor would reject and examples that he would favor.
11. How can technical and professional interpretations of nursing obscure its moral sense? How is it possible for nurses to be professionally and technically competent and still recognize nursing's moral sense?
12. How can Marx's interpretation of compassion and Taylor's interpretation of authenticity help unite Noddings's natural caring and ethical caring into a call to compassionate authentic care?

REFERENCES

Bishop, Anne H. and John R. Scudder, Jr. (1990). *The practical, moral, and personal sense of nursing: A phenomenological philosophy of practice*. Albany, NY: State University of New York Press.

Bishop, Anne H. and John R. Scudder, Jr. (1991). *Nursing: The practice of caring*. Sudbury, MA: National League for Nursing, Jones and Bartlett Publishers.

Carpenito, Linda J. (1995). *Nursing diagnosis: Application to clinical practice* 6th ed. Philadelphia: J. B. Lippincott.

Chinn, Peggy. (1994). Foreword. In M. E. Lashley, M. T. Neal, E. T. Slunt, L. M. Berman, and F. H. Hultgren. *Being called to care* (pp. vii–viii). Albany, NY: State University of New York Press.

Fry, Sara T. (1989). Toward a theory of nursing ethics. *Advances in Nursing Science*, 11:4, 9–22.

Fry, S. T. and Veatch, R. M. (2000). *Case Studies in Nursing Ethics* 2nd edition. Boston, MA: Jones & Bartlett.

Gadow, Sally. (1980). Existential advocacy: Philosophical foundation of nursing. In Stuart F. Spicker & Sally Gadow (Eds.), *Nursing: Images and ideals*. New York: Springer.

Heidegger, Martin. (1962). *Being and time*. trans. J. Macquarrie & E. Robinson. New York: Harper and Row.

Holy Bible, Revised Standard Version.

James, William. (1948). The moral philosopher and the moral life. In A. Castell (Ed.), William James, *Essays in pragmatism*. New York: Hafner Press.

James, William. (1958). *Talks to teachers on psychology: And to students on some of life's ideals*. New York: W. W. Norton.

Lashley, Mary Ellen, Maggie T. Neal, Emily Todd Slunt, Louise M. Berman, and Francine H. Hultgren. (1994). *Being called to care*. Albany, NY: State University of New York Press.

Marx, Werner. (1992). *Toward a phenomenological ethics: Ethos and the life-world*. Albany, NY: State University of New York Press.

Orem, Dorothea E. (1985). *Nursing: Concepts of practice* (3rd ed.). New York: McGraw Hill.

Pellegrino, E. (1985). The caring ethic. In A. H. Bishop and J. R. Scudder, Jr. (Eds.), *Caring, curing, coping: Nurse, physician, patient relationships* (pp. 8–30). University, AL: University of Alabama Press.

Taylor, C. (1991). *The ethics of authenticity*. Cambridge, MA: Harvard University Press.

Chapter 6

The Ethical in Holistic Practice

Holistic care enframes both technical and basic care in an ethic of caring. In holistic care, the ethical is an integral aspect of practice. In fact, it is often difficult to distinguish the ethical from the practical in holistic care. In this chapter, with the help of Richard Zaner, we will show that the ethical can be discerned from the merely practical in an ethics of practice. We will also show that ethics can contribute to nursing practice directly by helping nursing fulfill the moral intent of nursing practice.

Zaner's Clinical Ethics

Zaner's (1988) clinical ethics for medicine has much to offer nursing ethics. Through the years, we have worked closely with Zaner and have frequently discussed with him the implications of his clinical ethics for nursing ethics. Our purpose in considering Zaner's clinical ethics is to gain insight and understanding that will contribute to developing an ethics of practice appropriate to nursing rather than to give an adequate interpretation of his ethics.

Zaner, in developing his clinical ethics, rejects the assumption of most traditional ethics that a moral person is primarily an autonomous, detached, rational decision maker. This approach, he contends, is based on two questionable assumptions. First, the self is self-contained, insulated from others, and has only its own thoughts and feelings. Second, other persons are not experienced directly but are inferred from sensory experiences of the other's body (Zaner, 1988). Zaner rejects both assumptions. He contends that human beings, rather than being isolated and insulated, develop by mutuality and shared relationships. The moral life, rather than being an autonomous, rational application of abstract principles, is essentially mutual and communal. Whereas Zaner has shown how the detached, rational, autonomous approach does not make sense in medical practice, we have shown in previous work that it does not make sense in nursing practice.

> Nurses know that the above assumptions are unsound from their own experience. If the self is autonomous, in that it is closed in on itself, and therefore unable to grasp another person's meaning directly, nursing as practiced would be impossible. If a nurse can only infer meaning from a person's bodily movement rather than grasp the meaning from the body's expressiveness, nursing practice would certainly have to be altered. Imagine trying to turn a patient on a bed with efficiency and care to avoid unnecessary suffering if each grimace, body tension, grunt and moan, was to be taken as a sign from which to infer what was going on inside the body and then be correlated to the appropriate technique inferred from each sign. Instead, most nurses immediately recognize what the patient's bodily expressions mean and move him appropriately, drawing on long years of practical experience. (Bishop & Scudder, 1990, pp. 125–126).

Zaner not only shows why traditional ethics is not suited for clinical situations, he develops an ethic appropriate for clinical situations. He contends that such an ethics would have to meet three requirements.

ZANER'S REQUIREMENTS FOR A CLINICAL ETHICS

1. The work of ethics requires strict focus on the specific situational definition of each involved person.
2. Moral issues are presented solely within the contexts of their actual occurrence.
3. The situational participants are the principal resources for the resolution of the moral issues presented.*

From these three requirements, Zaner develops a clinical ethics that works on behalf of all participants in the situation, including those who receive care (patients, families, friends), the caregivers (physicians, nurses, and others), and the caregiving institution and its civic and social supporters. Such an ethics requires good communication between the participants, especially skill in listening to clients and using language that is easily understood. Good communication requires skilled probing to determine what is bothering those involved and how they understand their situation. The goal of communication is to help people make their own decisions concerning care and treatment based upon their beliefs and values.

---

*From *Ethics and the Clinical Encounter* (p. 243–244+) by Richard Zaner, 1988, Englewood Cliffs, NJ: Prentice Hall.

The Ethical in Holistic Practice   87

For Zaner, clinical ethics is primarily concerned with enablement rather than with providing authoritative solutions to moral problems. Those involved in health care situations are the resources necessary to enable all involved to reach satisfactory solutions and adequate regimens of care. They are the ones who will have to live with the consequences of their decisions and actions. For Zaner, enablement is "that communicative process whereby situational participants are provided with the understanding, the means, opportunities, power, or authority, already intrinsic to their situation, to effect change by their decisions" (Zaner, 1988, p. 248).

Zaner places health care ethics within the context of the clinical situation rather than within the context of traditional philosophical ethics. Those of us who believe that health care ethics should begin with the inherent moral sense of practice favor this move. However, we believe that nursing ethics can better be articulated as an ethics of practice. We came to the conclusion that an ethics of practice is appropriate for nursing through our many years of interpreting nursing as a practice with an inherent moral sense. Reading and interpreting Zaner's descriptions of his practice as an ethicist in his book, *Troubled Voices: Stories of Ethics and Illness* (1993), generated new insights into the meaning and appropriateness of an ethics of practice for nursing.

The case that especially enlightened our interpretation of an ethics of practice for nursing was one recommended by Zaner that takes place in a medical context but speaks as forcefully to nursing ethics as to medical ethics.

> Recently I received a call from a physician who wanted me to stop by to see a young man who had been hospitalized and was refusing hemodialysis. Refusal of treatment meant death. The patient was in his late twenties, and he had been hospitalized numerous times the previous summer for all manner of problems and was apparently just fed up with everything. . . .
>
> He had been born with spina bifida, making him paraplegic and hydrocephalic, and had a surgically implanted shunt that took the cerebral-spinal fluid from his brain to his abdomen. . . .
>
> That summer he had began [sic] to suffer from severe diarrhea, dehydration, infections, and a malfunctioning bladder and was repeatedly hospitalized. As if all that were not enough, his kidneys had begun to fail and he had become anemic. Now, hospitalized again, he staunchly refused to have dialysis even though it held the promise of at least some benefit, even a return to home and possibly the job he had held for some years. His physician, thinking that the young man was experiencing depression, prescribed an antidepressant hoping that he might, in a less distressed state, change his mind. . . .
>
> But despite the antidepressant, he continued to refuse dialysis. Within a few days, the poisons inevitably built up and dialysis was seriously needed. His mother was terrified. His physician had gone out of town for the weekend and the resident and nurses seemed at loggerheads with this patient's persistent refusal.

In the press of circumstances, the physician covering for the attending decided to have a psychiatrist assess his competence. Surely, it was thought, no one in his right mind would refuse treatments that promised relief and return to normalcy. Unsurprisingly, by that time the psychiatrist found him "temporarily incompetent," and his "decision against dialysis" was taken to be a function of depression and failing thought processes, said to be caused by the build-up of poisons in his bloodstream. Armed with that, the covering physician was able to place the catheter and take him off to be dialyzed.

When the attending returned he was quite concerned—furious is probably more accurate. Not only had his patient been dialyzed despite refusing it the previous week, but here the young man was alert once again—the dialysis had, after all, done its thing—and very disturbed at being forced to have dialysis. In fact, he continued his adamant refusal of any further sessions with the dialysis machine. Both the attending and his mother were in a bind: both wanted to respect what they considered to be the young man's competently expressed refusal though knowing that dialysis was actually beneficial. But he said that he had had enough; in fact a lifetime of enough. . . .

I came back to see Tom and his mother. . . . We moved directly to the issues at hand. Did he understand the implications of his refusal of dialysis? In a way, he did; but as we talked it seemed to me that he hadn't thought it out at all well. He was in fact behaving rather differently than one would expect when meeting someone firmly refusing potentially life-saving treatment. It's not that he was calmly accepting. He had not in fact discussed the matter with his mother; he had not really even thought about it much for himself. He had not signed any advanced directive; the idea hadn't even occurred to him. And his mother had not raised the issue with him of the advanced directive or the clear consequence of his refusal. The thought that he would die without dialysis had, so to speak, sort of sidled past his awareness now and then, but he had not confronted matters squarely. . . .

Trying to learn more about Tom personally, I asked him about his job, one which he obviously enjoyed and in which he took some pride. It was an office-type position with a state agency, and it had given him a good deal of independence. Before he became so sick some months ago, he had even started to think he could get his own apartment and begin to live on his own. *That*, it seemed to me, was what was really on his mind. The numerous illnesses and hospitalizations had eventually required him to quit his job, which more than anything else seemed the source of his depression. Like all of us at one time or another, he had it all "figured out": on dialysis he would not be able to hold a job, much less go back to the one he really liked—*ergo*, life ain't worth it, so let's just give up. Being "normal," working and living independently, had become an insurmountable goal when viewed from his perspective.

He continued talking and I listened. A few months ago, he said, almost as an afterthought, he had been told by his supervisor that his job would be waiting for him when he was able to return. As soon as he said this he noticeably perked up; his talk became more lively, his gestures more animated.

"That's right," his mother quickly affirmed, "Mrs. Y did say you could have your job back when you're able."

"But how can I work," Tom's tremulous words seemed at once hopeful and wary, "when I've got to be on that damned machine so much?"

His mother and I vied with each other to get the thing said: work was indeed possible. Hadn't he discussed this with his doctor? He wasn't sure. Perhaps he had been so wrapped up in grief and a deep sense of loss that he hadn't heard. Or perhaps none of his doctors had thought to mention it, or if any of them had, Tom hadn't understood. In any event, it was clear that the way things appeared had changed dramatically for him. I suggested that he really needed to find out much more about dialysis and to call up his supervisor to check with her about returning to work. . . . It was perfectly obvious that he did not want to refuse dialysis and that he desperately wanted to get out of the hospital and back to work. . . .

The last time I visited Tom he was on the dialysis machine. He told me that his boss had told him that he could have his old job back. He was very upbeat, joshing about the machine, joking with his nurse, and offering to come to one of my classes and talk about himself.*

In reconsidering this clinical encounter, Zaner was haunted by a series of questions. "When Tom first expressed his refusal to undergo dialysis, shouldn't that have had priority? Did his decline into renal psychosis change the competency with which he chose that condition? The decline, after all, was exactly what one would expect to occur. Within a day or so, he would have lapsed into an irreversible coma and then died. And wasn't this just what he had chosen?" (Zaner, 1993, p. 54) Had it not been for a fortuitous lack of communication between two physicians, his decision would have been honored, his rights respected, and he would have died.

Tom, however, had chosen to forego treatment without adequate knowledge of how dialysis would affect his life, especially his job and his desire to be more independent. Those who discussed this matter with Tom did so in the context of to-treat or not-to-treat and of Tom's *right* to deny treatment if competent. But why had no one inquired about the reason for his despondency and feeling of hopelessness? Zaner, called in as an ethicist, did inquire, but why hadn't Tom's physician or nurse done so? Why had they limited their concern to whether or not to give the dialysis that would make his continued

---

*From *Troubled Voices: Stories of Ethics and Illness* (pp. 47–55) by Richard M. Zaner, 1993, Cleveland, Ohio: Pilgrim Press. Used with permission.

living possible? Why had they not, as Zaner did, helped him discover what would make his life meaningful enough to endure dialysis? Tom knew well the suffering and limitations of a life dependent on medicine and others. As he says, "He had had a lifetime of enough!" Therefore, his refusal of dialysis did not result from being of unsound mind, but of not knowing his own mind. He needed to discover what would make a dialysis-dependent life worth living. Zaner, by entering his life-world, helped him to make the discovery that restored him to mental health, physical health, and the moral good for his life.

Ethics is a part of, rather than apart from, health care practice for Zaner. This is evident in his comments concerning Tom.

> We sense how deeply Tom felt torn away from what he had most wanted to be, compellingly pulled to keep alive his hope for independence even while he thought it was lost, as dead as he thought he now wanted to be. But it was not death, but a particular way of being alive that he most wanted (Zaner, 1993, p. 142).

For Zaner, medical practice is not limited to bodily functions fostered by chemical and surgical interventions; it also concerns the well-being of the whole person considered in light of that person's medical situation. For Zaner, ill persons like Tom find themselves faced "with a basic challenge to their sense of self. What and who we are, what we hope to be and become, even whether we will continue to be at all, is in one way or another at stake in these circumstances. This poses basic moral questions" (Zaner, 1993, p. 137). For Zaner, then, moral issues are posed by facing the problem of our own being and becoming in light of illness or debilitation and possible treatments to alleviate them. An ethicist helps persons place their illness, debilitation, and treatment within the context of patients's being and becoming as expressed in their beliefs and values.

People usually do not reflect on their basic beliefs and values in everyday living. Illness, debilitation, and treatment call forth such reflection. Working with an ethicist becomes the occasion for difficult, disquieting, and insightful reflection (Zaner, 1993, p. 147). Zaner believes that the ethicist's job is to help patients face philosophical issues inherent to their medical situation rather than to function as an expert who instructs patients on making moral decisions using traditional ethical procedures and norms. By exploring possible actions in light of beliefs and values in a clinical context, Zaner hopes to help people reach their own decisions. These decisions often emerge with sudden clarity.

> When the dialysis patient, Tom, for instance, began talking about his job and his hopes of getting an apartment, a veritable transformation took place in his gestures and words. I could almost see a light bulb go on. He was suddenly enlivened, talking about how he would get back to work, get an apartment. Yet only a moment before, he had been muted, his gestures slow and heavy, his voice and words softened by sadness, grief, loss. (Zaner, 1993, p. 149)

Zaner believes that clinical ethics helps people to come to "Ah-ha!" experiences that bring into focus how what is important in their lives relates to their health care.

For Zaner, an ethicist creates a caring relationship in which decisions are made in the context of being cared for and being treated with respect. These relationships are created by affiliation and compassion. In a relationship of affiliation, the ethicist reaches out to others in order to see their situation from their point of view. In a relationship of compassion, the ethicist enters into a relationship of "feeling-with-others" (Zaner, 1993, p. 146).

For Zaner, the moral sense of health care is not only evident in his ethics but is constitutive of it. He affirms the integral relation between ethics and health care practice that often is obscured by viewing ethics as an adjunct activity to medical and nursing practice. Those who hold the adjunct view believe that ethics is needed to resolve moral problems that are tangential to practice. Rather than arguing directly for an integral relationship between ethics and practice, Zaner discloses it by interpreting well-chosen examples. His disclosure of the ethical import of the cases he considers evokes in his readers a moral concern for the ill. Rather than the traditional opposition between the detachment of traditional ethics and the caring presence of practice, Zaner's ethical practice expresses his concern for the well-being of the ill and how ethicists can foster that well-being. His ethical practice is directed at fostering the patient's well-being. He describes that practice and articulates its meaning in a way that enhances the ethicist's ability and commitment to foster the well-being of the patient.

After listening to us read a paper on ethics of practice in which we featured the case of Tom, a family practice physician stated that he had difficulty determining how ethics could be distinguished from good practice. He contended that any good physician would do what Zaner did. He apparently expected us to disagree with him. When we agreed with him, he wanted to know what made ethics distinct from general medical care and why an ethicist would be needed in medicine. He seemed to think that an ethicist is a specialist who could be called in to "take over" moral problems, much the way an oncologist would be called in when cancer was suspected. Zaner finds being called an ethicist in this context amusing. When his philosophical colleagues asked him what he has become, he says with a wry smile, "I am an ethicist." Zaner's amusement stems from his belief that he is not a specialist in the sense that an oncologist is. Moral decisions are the most common and essential decisions human beings make. The family physician was right in contending that a good physician should help patients understand how treatments relate to their beliefs, values, and aspirations for the good life. From our conversation with him, we had no doubt that this was what he considered good medical practice. The fact that he had traveled from South Africa to the Netherlands to participate in a conference on the human sciences indicates that he was an unusual physician. He believed, as we do, that moral considerations are an essential part of practice. Therefore, he took it for granted that physicians would be concerned with helping patients make morally right decisions. Ethicists should not take over ethics in practice from health care professionals. Instead, they should help them recognize the ethical considerations inherent in practice and how to engage in ethics of practice more adequately.

Most nurses could have helped Tom discover what would have made an even more dependent life worth living. In fact, nurses are usually better situated and prepared by experience, education, and disposition than most physicians to be involved in an ethics of practice. Nursing practice involves ethical considerations with which most nurses are capable of dealing. They may need help from an ethicist to prepare them to recognize the moral aspects of nursing care and to assist them with especially difficult cases. Most cases in nursing ethics books focus on exceptionally difficult cases, but most moral decisions made by nurses concern issues that do not require the assistance of ethicists to resolve. Nurses need to be taught to recognize and articulate these issues as moral ones. One major function of ethicists is to disclose the moral in health care situations, as Zaner does in his recent book (1993).

Because Zaner primarily discloses the ethical in medical practice, we will attempt such disclosure in cases involving nursing care. Often the ethical in nursing care is disclosed in relationships of caring presence with patients in extremely difficult situations. These cases concern how to care in difficult situations rather than how to solve difficult moral problems. Nurse Robin Kramer tells the story of Lara, relating how nurses reached out with compassion to her and her family and helped them live fully in the face of the young woman's impending death.

"Lara, as I intuitively expected, was a bright-eyed, blond fourteen-year-old girl who, despite her illness, managed to smile and show a spunky personality at our first meeting. She was trying to be brave, but the fear in her eyes was undeniable. I introduced myself as the pediatric oncology clinical nurse specialist and began to orient Lara and her family to the Medical Center of the University of California at San Francisco. I explained that my role was to inform them about diagnostic tests that would occur over the next few days, to educate them about the disease and treatment once the diagnosis was confirmed, to coordinate Lara's medical and nursing care, to act as a liaison to the medical staff, fielding concerns and grievances, to help in any way possible, and to just be a friend during this frightening experience.

"I assured Lara and her family that although UCSF is a large medical center, Lara's care would be individualized. She would not be just 'another patient' or 'a case study' to us, but a very important person. She and her family would be the focus of our care. I also reassured the family that because UCSF is a large medical center, we have access to the latest knowledge and technology.

"Over the next two days, while waiting for confirmation of the diagnosis, I did a lot of listening. I heard about the symptoms and events that had led to Lara's hospitalization. I listened to the expression of shock, fear, and guilt—how could this diagnosis of leukemia be possible? The nursing staff and I spent considerable time getting to know Lara and her family—their coping strengths, their weaknesses, who supports whom and how. We did not negate their concerns or try to offer false assurance. We acknowledged their feelings as real and helped the family sort through them in a healthy and meaningful way.

"It was clear to all involved that one of the most useful things we could do for this distraught family, who was in a strange and overwhelming place, was to assist them, little by little, in gaining control over their experiences. This involved helping them anticipate and be prepared for what was to come, for how it might feel or look physically and emotionally. It also involved helping them to continue in their usual roles as much as possible and engaging them as appropriate in the decisions affecting Lara's care. The sincerity conveyed to the family convinced them that someone would always be there for them during the low times."

Robin and the nursing staff structured Lara's care to meet her concerns during her eight weeks of hospitalization. They secured a telephone for her so that she could call her friends. Robin followed Lara's lead in providing care: sometimes they joked, sometimes listened to music, and at other times they talked about serious issues. Robin nonverbally indicated to Lara that it was all right to be angry or depressed. Robin and the staff arranged a birthday party for Lara, and Robin took Lara and two friends on a Sunday outing in her car.

In spite of medical treatment and nursing care, Lara's prognosis continued to grow dimmer. When Lara and her family considered a bone marrow transplant (BMT), her nurses arranged for a young woman who had had a BMT to come to talk to Lara. In discussing the possibilities of a BMT with Lara and her family, Robin did not temper their enthusiasm with the negative side of BMT. When there was no match for BMT within the family, Robin took the opportunity to explain the unpleasant side of BMT and acknowledge the gamut of emotions evoked when certain decisions are out of one's control.

The ability to control Lara's condition lessened. Lara started to have high fevers, seemed tired despite transfusions, and needed oxygen. At Robin's suggestion, Lara's mother called the family together to be with Lara in her final hours.

"Lara needed to be intubated because her respiratory status continued to deteriorate. This was a terrible experience for her; she continuously gestured to us to remove the tube. The medical and nursing staff, along with Lara's family, acknowledged that Lara's death was imminent. Our greatest gift to Lara would be to give back her dignity by removing the respirator. She immediately started talking in a high, squeaky voice, and plans quickly developed to have a party 'to toast Lara's awakening,' as Joann aptly described it.

"As I visited with Lara, she looked me directly in the eyes and said, 'I'm so sick, am I going to die?' Although it was a matter of seconds before I answered, it seemed like hours as my mind groped for the right words. I did not avert my gaze and answered from my heart: 'I'm frightened Lara, you are so sick that you could die. I know you must be terribly scared, too. Everyone you love is with you, and we won't leave.'

She nodded and quietly closed her eyes to rest. Shortly thereafter, the champagne arrived, and we toasted Lara—her extubation, her courage, and her spirit. She smiled and said, 'I love you all very much.' " Two hours later, she died peacefully with her family nearby.*

Robin not only cared for Lara but for her family as well. Her mother commented, "Any degree of stability I was able to maintain over the next eight weeks was due largely to the unwavering support and encouragement of this dedicated young woman. Her daily concern was not only for the patient but for each family member" (Benner & Wrubel, 1989, p. 304).

The foregoing is an example of both excellent practice and ethical care in that the values of the patient and the response of the nurse to those values are integrally involved in patient care. The response of Robin—indeed the whole health care staff—to Lara's situation was one of affiliation and compassion. The way the nurses responded to Lara's situation made evident the moral sense that often goes unnoticed in health care. In this case, recognition of the moral sense was not the result of a major ethical decision. The only major decision in Lara's care concerned removing the respirator. Yet, in the story, this decision was simply the continuation of a pervasive, ongoing way of caring for Lara that helped her to live her last days as fully as possible. Everyday moral decisions included making arrangements for her to phone her friends, arranging a birthday party for her, and making special arrangements for a trip with some of her friends. Some of the contributions of nurses to Lara's living as fully as possible were mentioned after her death by her mother: one nurse braided Lara's hair to prevent baldness; another nurse attempted to take her to a concert and, when that was not possible, brought her a full report and memorabilia from the concert; another shared her tapes with Lara and talked with her about the music Lara liked (Benner & Wrubel, 1989, pp. 303–306).

Discovering the way fourteen-year-olds want to live the remainder of their lives rarely comes from philosophical discussions of the meaning of life. In Lara's case, it came from her nurses, especially from Robin's being with her and discovering what gave meaning to her life: conversing with friends, listening to music, escaping from the hospital, having parties, being attractive, and, above all, being surrounded by caring people who loved her and whom she loved. Lara's nurses disclosed to Lara and her family that their care *of* her expressed their care *for* her.

Another example of such care is evident in the home care given by Barbara to a man whose situation was quite different from Lara's. He seemed to have little to live for, having lost his wife, his twin brother, his business, and his independence. Now, facing the loss of his health from congestive heart failure and his dependence on continuous nursing care, he felt that his life had little meaning.

---

*From *The Primacy of Caring: Stress and Coping in Health and Disease* (pp. 298–302) by Patricia Benner and Judith Wrubel, 1989, Menlo Park, CA: Addison-Wesley. Used with permission of Robin Kramer.

One day, upon one of my home visits as I was assessing him and engaging him in conversation, he began to cry again. Having built a rapport with him and feeling I had gained his trust, I put down my stethoscope, got down on my knees by the side of his chair and took his hand in mine.... I knelt there holding his hand and quietly listening, and then I shared with him how much he had come to mean to me—that knowing him had enriched my life—that he was a very special person. A bond was forged that day. A bond of trust, understanding, and caring. It is a bond that continues to grow as I continue to care for this patient with all of those losses and chronic needs that impact his daily life.

What struck me the most was that it was not my stethoscope, or my teaching that impacted him the most, but simply *time*—time to talk, to touch, and to care.

In the preceding case, the relationship of practice and morality is so intertwined that it is difficult to separate one from the other. The nurse discovered that her patient's well-being required much more than ordinary assessment and care. In dialogue, she realized that her patient's emptiness emerged from the loss of everything that gave his life meaning and a sense of worth. Her personal way of being with him helped restore meaning and worth to his life.

Barbara's personal relationship with her patient was enhanced by meeting him on his level; recall that she knelt down beside him in his chair. Kay Toombs (1992), a philosopher with multiple sclerosis, tells how posture and speech affect ill and debilitated persons. She is irritated by people who ignore her by directing questions to her husband and referring to her in the third person when she is in a wheelchair: "Would *she* like to sit at this table?" "What would *she* like to drink?" (p. 65). Toombs recounts how, on one occasion when she was wheeled up to a security barrier in an airport, an attendant turned to her husband and asked, "Can *she* walk at all?" Her husband retorted, "Yes, and she can talk, too!" (136). Toombs contends that autonomy is directly related to the ability to assume an upright posture. She says, "To be able to 'stand on one's own two feet' is of more than figurative significance" (p. 65). Toombs asserts how demeaning some spatial terms used to refer to the ill can be.

There is more than metaphorical significance to such expressions as "to look down on," and "to look up to." In the hospital setting the patient, more often than not, is in bed and must "look up to" the doctor who "stands" talking and "looking down on" the patient. In "looking up to" the doctor, and "being looked down on," the patient feels on an unequal "footing" with the physician, concretely diminished in autonomy.... In this regard it is worth noting that patients are likely to feel much less "inferior" if the physician sits down by the bedside, so that they are on the same level ("eye to eye") when communicating with one another. (Toombs, 1992, pp. 65–66)

The way in which nurses posture themselves in relationship to patients and speak of their lived spatial relationships with them is of ethical import. Posture and speech can deny or assure patients of their autonomy, and make evident the extent of their nurse's concern for them and involvement with them.

In the foregoing cases, both Barbara and Robin established a relationship with their patients that fostered their well-being and enhanced their zest for life. In both cases, being compassionately called to care by the plight of another person appears to be more important than exceptional nursing skill or knowledge. Using such cases to illustrate the meaning of nursing ethics has the danger of reinforcing an unfortunate misunderstanding of the meaning of the moral in nursing. It can imply that morality in nursing concerns "going the extra mile" outside of and detached from nursing care. In both of the above cases, the nurses "go the extra mile," but in a direction called for by excellent nursing practice. Expressed another way, both nurses fulfill the moral sense of nursing by moving beyond competent care to excellent care in order to foster their patient's well-being.

An example of nursing ethics that is less concerned with "going the extra mile" in personal relations and that involves the integral relationship of moral, personal, technical, and practical care is the case of Mr. Jones. In this example, his nurse, Mary Cucci, skillfully restored Mr. Jones to his lived body after he had lost the ability to live in and through his body because of fear resulting from the repeated firings of an implanted defibrillator and from cardiac arrests.

> "The night of his admission, . . . he had been 'automatically' defibrillated twenty times in the period of an hour before an intravenous medication could control the rhythm.
>
> "I first met Mr. Jones the morning after his admission to the CCU. The nurse on the previous shift told me about the terror he had been through. He had screamed with the repeated defibrillation, had required a significant amount of sedation, and had been rambling and panicky until the sedation took effect.
>
> "As I entered the room, . . . his eyes focused on me, but the rest of his body seemed frozen in the bed. His body was limp and his muscles looked wasted as if he had lost considerable weight. We had a brief, quiet conversation of introduction. . . . I told him that I understood that he had been through a great deal. I asked him gently if he would tell me how he felt about it. He replied: 'How would you feel? It was a nightmare.' As he continued to speak, his face began to reflect his pain and anxiety. His eyes began to tear. His voice was tremulous and frail. . . . 'What am I going to do now? I thought this (the implanted defibrillator) was the last answer. What if it happened again? I couldn't stand that'. . . . I told him that I would help him find some answers, and that I was going to help him through this. I shared my impressions of him; that he appeared overwhelmed, with a million thoughts running

through his mind at once, and that he seemed to feel as if he felt out of control. He said, 'Yes, that is how I feel.' He seemed surprised that somehow I understood. He also talked about feeling betrayed by the device that was supposed to be the answer. He talked about his fear of it happening again. I discussed Mr. Jones's distress with his physicians and encouraged them to discuss the possibility of turning off the defibrillator while he was in the CCU. By two in the afternoon, with Mr. Jones's approval, the defibrillator was turned off. . . .

"Despite the emotional and intellectual intensity he displayed, Mr. Jones moved minimally in the bed. This intense man appeared trapped in a frozen shell. Some of it was due to the debilitation of his weight loss and recent illnesses, but as I began talking to him about moving more and maintaining and building his physical strength, I began to realize he was afraid to move. He admitted it. Apparently, several of his tachycardias had occurred during exertion. This time I persisted and after an explanation of the importance of moving his arms, legs, and body gently around in the bed, he began to make some progress. Suddenly he was aware of every premature heartbeat he had. I told him when he was right and when he was wrong. We watched the monitor together. We set up a plan for increased mobility and negotiated each limit. I stayed with him through each new step. It was like watching someone wake up physically, but the process was slower and more obviously sequential. It was the mental hurdle we were really facing. I challenged him to meet the goals we set. I distracted him with conversation. He watched the clock ferociously and met his goal with not a minute extra given. He began moving more in the bed without thinking about it. More of his body participated as he continued to talk of the intense emotional issues he faced. I teased him, conjoled him, and danced with him as he transferred to the chair. I challenged him more each day and ignored his fake whine when he half-heartedly pleaded abuse. It became a joke. He learned to monitor his pulse to guide his activity progression. This was a long, slow process of building belief in himself. I told him throughout that I knew it was difficult, that I admired his strength, and that I knew he could do it."

Through dialogue with Mr. Jones, Mary discovered that he had never really confronted the likelihood of his own death and that he had lived a life that was so ordered that he even followed a diagram for each day's work. Now he could not plan or order his life and was confronted with the fear of death. He commented, "This time everything has been taken away," to which Mary responded that his wife, who had faithfully supported him, had not been taken away. He responded, "If it wasn't for her, I don't know what I would do."

"Several months after discharge, Mr. Jones and his wife returned to the CCU to say hello. We greeted each other with hugs and smiles. He had gained weight and I teased him about his potbelly. Eight months after discharge he is still doing well and reports to his physician that he is feeling better and better."

The goal of nursing practice is to foster the well-being of the patient, and, thus, it is to fulfill the moral sense of health care. Ethics is concerned with how well the moral sense is fulfilled. In the preceding story, Mary helps foster the well-being of Mr. Jones by engrossment in his situation and with dialogue that assures him that his response to his illness and treatment is understandable and acceptable, and that she is willing to act on his behalf. She shares Mr. Jones's fears with his physician, and they agree, with Mr. Jones's permission, to terminate the defibrillator. This measure leads him to face his own mortality and to raise the question of whether or not he is committing suicide. Because Mary feels inadequate to deal with this question, she refers Mr. Jones to a chaplain for consultation. She also seeks the assistance of a psychiatric nurse to help him deal with the disruptions in his life that he is so ill-prepared to handle. She personally helps him to understand that his relationship with his wife is a source of meaning and assurance. Perhaps her greatest contribution is the tactful, resourceful, and compassionate way in which she helps him overcome his fear of bodily movement and her skill, sensitivity, and persistence in helping him learn to relive his body within the constraints of new circumstances.

The fearful response of Mr. Jones to his situation shows us how illness can alienate us from our body and how it can restrict our space. Mr. Jones was literally afraid to move and was virtually imprisoned in a strange body that he feared. He could not move because of fear that movement would trigger tachycardia. Although his fear was exaggerated, it was not unwarranted. He had to learn bodily movement because his physical well-being required movement. Mary helped him learn to move in ways that overcame his fear by using a monitor. It is important, however, to recognize that he was not learning to move according to the monitor, but according to his lived experience of his body. The monitor merely gave him assurance and set limits that were recognized by the lived body. Eventually, he was able to move within these limits, even when Mary deliberately distracted him from being overtly conscious of his body.

ETHICS IN HOLISTIC CARE

Mary contributed to his physical well-being by fostering the movement that his body required to heal. To do this, she worked with his lived body. He had to learn to relive his body, not just for his physical well-being, but for his personal well-being. Toombs (1992) observes that "to address the patient's experiences of disorder, attention must be paid not only to the physical mani-

---

From *The Primacy of Caring: Stress and Coping in Health and Illness* (pp. 247–250) by Patricia Benner and Judith Wrubel, 1989, Menlo Park, CA: Addison-Wesley. Used with permission of Mary Cucci.

festation of a disease state but also to the changing relations between body, self, and world" (p. 82). She contends that chronic illness in particular requires giving attention to "essential features" of "embodiment . . . such as being-in-the-world, bodily intentionality, . . . body image, gestural display" and lived space and time (p. 82). These aspects of embodiment are evident in Mr. Jones's case. How can he be in a world in which everything is not controlled and he is not autonomous? His former bodily intentionality presupposed an ordered world in which his lived body functioned autonomously and reliably. His image of his body had to undergo a major transformation from that of control, order, and autonomy to a body subject to natural forces over which he had little control. His gestural display, rather than being one of power and self-assurance, became one of fear, uncertainty, and withdrawal. His space, which once was open and invited autonomous movement, had become not only confined to a bed, but to a strange body. He seemed to have no future because he could not project himself beyond the body into which he had retreated. Then Mary taught him how to live that body again. Instead of being a frightened stranger confined to a body that he occupied in fear, he once again became confidently embodied in the world.

When he returned several months later and greeted and hugged Mary, Mr. Jones's gestural display was that of a fully embodied person reaching out to embrace those for whom he cared. Mary reported that eight months later he felt better and that his "amiodarone had been reduced and no significant arrhythmias recurred" (Benner, 1987, p. 1172). Strangely, she omitted that he seemed to have become an embodied person living well with self, others, and world.

One aspect of care deals with treatment that cures or improves bodily function: "amiodarone had been reduced and no significant arrhythmias recurred." This refers primarily to the body as a biological machine. Ethics is important to this aspect of health care to ensure that technology is enframed in its original moral intent—that is, for the good of the other. A second aspect concerns the lived body interacting with self, others, and world. Concern for the well-being of the lived body is the focus of the ethical in holistic practice. For example, Tom's physicians focused on the body object: dialysis will keep it alive. Zaner focused on the lived body and world by asking, "Why should Tom want to live or die?"

Mary did not overtly address the philosophical question Mr. Jones asked concerning whether a life that could not be strictly ordered and controlled was worth living. Instead, she answered this question practically with her care for him. She obviously believed, as did Mr. Jones after he recovered from his fears, that it is good to be embodied and live your body in relationship to self, others, and the world. Mary concretely engaged in an ethics of practice that restored Mr. Jones to his lived body in relationship to self, others, and world. She moved him from entombment in his body to timid movement and finally to dancing in restoring him to the world that he so obviously enjoyed *being* in during their last meeting. Mary's holistic care that fostered the well-being of

Mr. Jones's lived body in relationship to self, others, and world is an example of the ethics of practice.

There are two kinds of care. One is a mechanistic care that treats the anatomical body as a machine to be fixed and controlled with machines, chemicals, and surgery. The purpose of the implanted defibrillator was to regulate the functioning of Mr. Jones's heart. The machine's failure not only concerned the anatomical body, but Mr. Jones's lived body as well. The machine was not experienced by Mr. Jones as a failed heart regulator, but as pain that must cease. Mary engaged in an ethics of practice when she placed the mechanistic therapy within the context of the lived body by having the machine disconnected.

The second way of caring directly concerns how the body is lived in relationship to self, others, and world. Mary engaged in ethics directly when her care in practical ways helped Mr. Jones face and answer questions related to his illness and debilitation. Mr. Jones's anxiety about future pain focused his attention on his lived body's relationship to the self. How could he become confident and assertive when he was under the constant threat of pain? His apprehension about lack of order and autonomy focused his concern on his lived body's relationship to the world. How could he live the ordered life required in business when his lived body made his world unpredictable and unreliable? His recognition of the importance of his wife focused his concern on the importance of his lived body to others. How could he refuse to undergo the therapy needed to restore his health when his wife was so important to him and dependent upon him?

Ethics in nursing practice is focused on the lived world and how wellness, illness, debilitation, and treatment affect the lived body's relation to self, others, and the world. Ethics helps nurses foster the well-being of the whole person as he/she projects himself/herself in the world. By so doing, it keeps nursing focused on its primary and inherent moral purpose: fostering the well-being of the other and on the holistic care through which that purpose is fulfilled.

STUDY QUESTIONS

1. What does Zaner mean by *clinical ethics*? Do you agree with Anne and Jack that Zaner's clinical ethics can make an important contribution to an ethics of practice for nursing? Why or why not?
2. Drawing on the story of Tom, give an interpretation of an ethics of practice. If you had been Tom's nurse, how would you have engaged in ethics? Give an example of when you have engaged in ethics from your experience of nursing. If your experience is limited, give an imaginary example.
3. Why is the nursing care of Laura by Robin and other nurses an example of ethical care? Describe other examples of nursing care in which the

morality of nurses involved quality care in difficult situations, rather than difficult moral issues to be resolved.

4. What does the case of Barbara and the experience of Kay Toombs indicate about how the posture of nurses in relating to patients is involved in ethical care?
5. Discuss the ethical questions Mr. Jones and Mary faced in her nursing care of him. Why do Anne and Jack contend that Mary answered some of the questions practically rather than theoretically?
6. How does Kay Toombs's analysis of how illness changes relationships between lived body, self, others, and world enlighten what Mr. Jones is experiencing?
7. Describe how Mary helps Mr. Jones learn to relive his body. Give an example of how you have helped or might help patients learn to relive their bodies or some function of their bodies, such as grasping or walking.
8. Why does Mary's report that Mr. Jones felt "better and better" and that his "amiodarone had been reduced and no significant arrhythmias recurred" fail to do justice to her excellent care? Do you believe that nurses often fail to articulate the full ethical significance of their care? Why or why not?
9. What two kinds of care are treated by Jack and Anne? What is the ethical import of each? How are they related to each other? In which is ethical care most involved? Why?
10. When nursing care is holistic, why are ethical considerations an integral aspect of nursing care?

REFERENCES

Benner, Patricia, & Wrubel, Judith. (1989). *The primacy of caring: Stress and coping in health and disease*. Menlo Park, CA: Addison-Wesley.

Bishop, Anne H., & Scudder, John R., Jr. (1990). *The practical, moral, and personal sense of nursing: A phenomenological philosophy of practice*. Albany, NY: State University of New York Press.

Toombs, S. Kay. (1992). *The meaning of illness: A phenomenological account of the different perspectives of physician and patient*. Dordrecht: Kluwer Academic Publishers.

Zaner, Richard M. (1988). *Ethics and the clinical encounter*. Englewood Cliffs, NJ: Prentice Hall.

Zaner, Richard M. (1993). *Troubled voices: Stories of ethics and illness*. Cleveland, OH: Pilgrim Press.

Chapter

Reflexive Dialogue on Ethics and Nursing

Ethics is integrally related to nursing because nursing is a practice with an inherent moral sense. Nursing ethics attempts to articulate that moral sense, to assess its fulfillment, to explore new possibilities for its fulfillment, and to appraise its moral adequacy. These articulations, appraisals, and explorations focus on nursing as practiced, especially on exemplars of nursing excellence. Exemplars both disclose the meaning of *good* nursing care and call nurses into relationships of holistic caring presence with patients.

In this work, we have interpreted nursing ethics in the five ways implied by the titles of the preceding five chapters. Chapter 2 investigated the meaning of being a good nurse by showing that care as practice and care as concern are integrally related to each other in good care. When nurses are attentive, efficient, and effective in their practice, they are being morally good persons because they are fulfilling the moral sense of nursing by fostering the well-being of patients. Being concerned about patient well-being is built into the practice and presupposed by it. Ethics not only contributes understanding of these two senses of good and how they relate to each other, but it also engages in critical appraisal of how well nursing fulfills its moral sense. This will become more evident in our dialogical interpretation of Betty, Trish, and Nancy as exemplars of a good nurse.

In Chapter 3, we described how nurses foster wholistic care by bringing together in an integral relationship medical care, specialized care, administrative support, and nursing care. We explored holistic care that goes beyond limiting care to *the* patient by recognizing and responding to the whole person. Margie's care for Mrs. Cooper disclosed the integral relationship between wholistic and holistic care, while Claire went beyond functioning as *the* nurse for *the* patient to integrate professional and personal care for a person suffering from terrible arthritis.

In Chapter 4, we attempted to describe caring presence drawing on Buber, Noddings, and Zaner. The relationship of ethics to caring presence is so evident that the ethical in nursing is often identified with caring presence. The reason for the tendency to identify the ethical in nursing with caring presence was apparent in the relationship of Beverly and Midori. Caring presence affirms the humanity of both nurse and patient and accords each the respect due a human being. It comforts and supports those cared for as they face suffering, treatment, and possible death, and, at the same time, it inspires and enlightens the care-giver.

In Chapter 5, we treated nursing as a calling by exploring the meaning of being called to care and philosophical interpretations that enlighten and heighten that call. We rejected the separation typical of Western thought in which call is thought of as motive divorced from meaning and practice. Then, with help from Chinn and Lashley, we showed that the call to care and the meaning of that care are integrally related to each other. Nursing ethics is concerned with understanding and evoking the call to care. Responding to that call is so built into nursing and to being a nurse that it is usually experienced as "Of course I will care." We discussed how Pellegrino restores the moral sense of call that is inherent in profession, and how James expands this calling to include responding to possibilities for the good that appear in our encounter with the world. We related how Jesus, through the story of the Good Samaritan, discloses how the plight of the neighbor calls nurses as human beings—as well as professionals—to care for those who need help. Finally, we combined Marx's ethics of compassion with Taylor's interpretation of an ethics of authenticity to show how the call to care can be situated in the meaning of being human.

In Chapter 6, with the help of Zaner's clinical ethics, we showed that nursing ethics is more adequately understood as an ethics of practice than as an applied philosophical ethics. The intent of both nursing ethics and nursing practice is to foster the well-being of the client. Ethics attempts to critique and foster fulfillment of the intent of nursing practice. Ethics has a limited involvement in that aspect of practice that is primarily technical and biological in that it only ensures that the technical fulfills its purpose of fostering the well-being of persons and that their rights are respected. Ethics is integrally involved in practice that concerns the lived body's relationship to self, others, world, and the life projects of persons. That ethics explores the relationship of illness and treatment to the lived body and personal projects is evident in Zaner's ethical care for Tom and in our interpretation of the case of Mary Cucci and Mr. Jones.

Although our approach to nursing ethics should be of interest to ethicists, our book is primarily intended for nurses and nursing students. Our purpose has not been to show how ethics can be applied to nursing. Instead, we have shown how the moral sense of nursing impacts nursing ethics. We want to make nurses aware of the moral import of their practice and how they can better fulfill its moral sense. We hope to encourage them to explore new possibilities by developing new ways to empower their care and by developing visions of the good that will direct their caring practice.

Helping nurses to recognize, fulfill, and enhance the moral sense of nursing requires getting down to cases. Consequently, we will conclude by exploring the meaning and implications for nursing ethics of the exemplars of being a good nurse, of wholistic and holistic care, of caring presence, and of an ethics of practice that we have previously discussed. Keeping with the exploratory nature of this interpretation, we will engage in a reflexive dialogue to disclose the meaning of each case for nursing ethics. Most of our writing comes from reflexive dialogue in which we attempt to ferret out the meaning of nursing, to place that meaning within a wider human context, and to explore new possibilities for enhancing nursing practice. We invite the reader to share in our reflexive dialogue.

Reflexive Dialogue

Anne: I always feel more adequate when I attempt to point out how the good is fostered in concrete nursing cases than when I attempt to justify calling what I do "nursing ethics."

Jack: You know how I feel about "Is this really X?" questions in philosophy. I remember when a young scholar challenged a leading phenomenologist by asking him if the paper he had read was *really* phenomenology. The philosopher responded, "I've never really thought about it, but I do work out of that tradition and I think I gave an adequate treatment of the philosophical issue with which I was concerned." Like him, I usually work out of a phenomenological tradition, and I am more concerned with how that tradition enlightens my understanding of the world than I am in how it fits into academic categories. In this book, I'm more concerned with articulating and fostering the good inherent in nursing practice than in answering the question, "Is what we're doing *really* ethics?"

Anne: Yes, but this is a book on nursing ethics, and we must be as clear as we can about what the stories we have included have to do with ethics.

Jack: I can hear some of my philosophical colleagues contending that the way we use and interpret examples tends to confuse morality with ethics. When I first studied ethics, we were taught that ethics concerns the theory of morality. Since my philosophical orientation has become more phenomenological, I have concluded that ethics is *thinking about the meaning of morality*. Consequently, nursing ethics concerns the meaning of being a morally good nurse.

Anne: Thinking about the meaning of good nursing requires interpreting the moral sense of nursing practice and examples of nurses who fulfill that sense.

Jack: Disclosing the meaning of morally good nursing through examples fits Paul Ricoeur's brief definition of phenomenology. He contends that phenomenology is a philosophy primarily concerned with disclosing meaning, that meaning is given as essence, and that essence is disclosed through well-chosen examples (Ricoeur, 1977). Interpretation helps clarify the meaning disclosed through examples and places them in a wider context of meaning.

Anne: But haven't we at times said that nurses were being ethical when they were concerned with being good nurses rather than with the meaning of being a good nurse?

Jack: Yes, we have. If you define ethics as articulating the meaning of being a good nurse, nurses often pursue the meaning of being a good nurse practically in the decisions they make concerning their care. Mary Cucci and Margie Smith actually did recognize and pursue the meaning of morally good nursing in their practice, even though they articulated it inadequately. One purpose of our book is to help nurses recognize and articulate the ethics of practice implicit in their care, hence our consideration of exemplars of morally good nursing and our interpretation of the moral sense of their practice.

On Being a Good Nurse

Anne: We entitled Chapter 2, "On Being a Good Nurse" because we wanted to explore the meaning of being a good nurse without talking about *the* nurse. The stories of Betty, Trish, and Nancy disclose different aspects of the meaning of being a good nurse, but all show the integral relationship between the sentiment and practice of care.

Jack: I found the story of Nancy bathing the patient especially intriguing. I'd never thought of bathing as a significant part of practice, but the way Nancy bathed her patient surely disclosed the moral sense of care. Her concern for her patient was so integrated into her practice that I was not aware of it until I reflected on it. Then I realized that she not only integrated concern for her patient's well-being in her sensitive care, but cared for her in a way that encouraged her to care for herself.

Anne: In the story of Trish, the moral sense of her care is so evident that we called it outstanding because it makes the moral sense of nursing stand out. When Trish couldn't get in touch with the physician, she reviewed the possible reasons that her patient had continued to be hypovolemic. When she decided that the reason could be hyperglycemia, she ordered a blood glucose level that was elevated to 600. Rather than playing it safe by waiting for the physician, her concern was first and foremost for the well-being of her patient.

Jack: Acting without official sanction, as Trish does, requires much courage. Betty showed the same kind of courage. Trish had a blood glucose level to indicate that her decision was the right one. Betty had to use her best judgment to change the regimen for her patient when she decided he needed sleep more than breathing exercises and chest physical therapy in the middle of the night. She reasoned that her patient, a young physician, needed a clear head to face the decisions he would have to make about his care. She was more concerned with fostering her patient's ability to direct his own life than with safely pursuing the agreed upon regimen.

WHOLISTIC AND HOLISTIC CARE

Anne: I know that many nurses will be asking where we found our definitions of *holistic* and *wholistic*.

Jack: Actually, we found it in nursing care. When we were asked by Lynn Rew, the editor of the *Journal of Holistic Nursing*, how to distinguish between *holistic* and *wholistic*, we began puzzling over it. Dictionaries were of no avail, nor were my philosophy colleagues. Then we discovered that holistic care had two different thrusts. One refers to nurses and patients responding to each other as whole persons rather than as objects placed in limiting professional or theoretical categories. The other has to do with creating whole care that has been separated by professional specialization and specialized theoretical study. We call care *wholistic* when disparate aspects have to be brought together in order to have whole care. In contrast, we speak of *holistic* care when care recognizes and fosters the wholeness of human experience in personal relationships between patient and nurse.

Anne: The differences between wholistic and holistic care are evident in Margie Smith's care for Mrs. Cooper. Her holistic care is evident in her being so engrossed in Mrs. Cooper's life situation that she recognizes that Mrs. Cooper's determination and courage outweigh the dismal prospects for prostheses for most persons of her age and health status. In her wholistic care, Margie goes to great lengths to foster the well-being of Mrs. Cooper. She engaged in a prolonged confrontation with the physician and the physical therapist. She elicited the help of occupational therapists, the clinical nurse specialist, and other staff nurses to prevent Mrs. Cooper's early discharge, to secure two new prostheses, and to arrange for the help necessary for her to learn to walk with them. This is an example of how wholistic and holistic care can foster patient well-being. It discloses the meaning of good nursing, but won't some ethicists question its inclusion in an ethics book?

Jack: The story of Margie and Mrs. Cooper should help nurses recognize excellent practice and call them to engage in good nursing care. Because nursing practice is designed to foster patient well-being, the reason for its inclusion seems obvious to me. But I realize that in this age of technical philosophy, some ethicists are apt to want more philosophical justification for inclusion of our exemplars in an ethics book. To question inclusion of a story that encourages moral excellence in an ethics book seems odd!

Anne: Margie is engaging in ethics by being Mrs. Cooper's existential advocate in the sense of Gadow's (1980) interpretation. She helps Mrs. Cooper discover and fulfill the meaning of her life in light of her illness, debilitation, and treatment.

Jack: By now, most nurses have some grasp of the meaning of Gadow's existential advocacy, but Margie extends the meaning of advocacy beyond Gadow. The further meaning of her advocacy, can be disclosed with an example. A friend of mine came to a lecture late and, not wanting to interrupt the proceedings, sat on the floor in the back of the meeting hall. Someone tapped him on the shoulder and said, "Would you be my advocate?" He turned and saw a man on crutches who immediately responded to his puzzled look by asking, "Would you help me find a seat?" Later the two discussed the meaning of advocacy, and the man with the crutches explained that an advocate is someone who helps you do what you cannot do without help, but does so in a way that liberates you from limitations imposed by your disability.

Anne: Margie fulfills that sense of advocacy. The moral sense of nursing pervades her advocacy of Mrs. Cooper. But I'm not sure that she explicitly recognizes the moral imperative inherent in nursing practice or that she realizes that nursing itself is constituted by that imperative. I am surprised that she sums up her outstanding care for Mrs. Cooper by saying, "I'm pleased that I was able to play an instrumental role in improving the quality of life for this patient," and that Margie regrets that she couldn't give a better example of "positive team-building." (See page 31.)

Jack: How can she say "an instrumental role" and "positive team-building?" "Instrumental role" implies technical proficiency rather than moral excellence. Her language blunts the moral impact of her forceful advocacy. Regardless of the adequacy of her language for conveying the moral sense of nursing, her care discloses it superbly. She is so intent on fostering Mrs. Cooper's well-being that she is willing to take on those who safely follow standard treatments for this type of patient rather than seeking treatment suited to Mrs. Cooper. Margie does this by building a team of defenders of the right who become advocates of Mrs. Cooper.

Anne: That sounds macho to me! As I remember it, Margie maneuvered through a web of connection and skillfully and sensitively encouraged others to see the right action. She persistently led others to the right action through wholistic care rather than, as you say, demanded that it be done as a right!

Jack: You're right. Her way of caring is well-described by Gilligan's feminist ethics. But do not miss the quality of her moral stance with concerns over whether it is feminine rather than masculine. She not only forcefully demands that nursing fulfill its moral sense, but also calls physicians and other health care workers to live up to a high standard of fostering the well-being of others. That's what is odd about her remark about not giving an example of positive team building. She builds a positive team out of a very unpromising situation.

Anne: It may seem odd to you that someone who is so practically and morally on target cannot articulate the meaning of her care, but not to me. Like many nurses, she has been taught to speak in technical and professional language rather than in the moral language common to everyday relationships. I've always felt that nurses were better moral beings than they give themselves credit for. Recently, the lack of recognition of the moral quality of our work has been obscured by the professional and technological language that was so evident in Margie's inadequate articulation of her excellent moral care.

Jack: Nurses not only fail to do justice to the moral quality of their practice, but they often focus on the wrong moral issues. For example, care and rights seem to me to go together. I'm puzzled by nursing scholars who foster unnecessary conflict between advocates of care and advocates of autonomy and rights.

Anne: You wouldn't be puzzled if you were a woman. Men have always taken advantage of the tendency of women to care and nurture. Although I believe—as you do—that care and rights go together, I can certainly understand why many of my colleagues are suspicious that emphasizing the value of caring might carry with it a denial of rights.

Jack: That's the reason we encountered so much opposition to our claim that one of the primary stances of nursing was the in-between stance in which nurses fostered unified care by bringing together nursing care, medical care, administrative and other assistance, family concerns and involvement, and the patient's desire for the good life. I remember how stunned I was by the vehemence of that opposition.

Anne: If we had thought through the positive meaning of that stance, we would have realized that it should be called *wholistic* care. I can't imagine a case that better shows how wholistic care fosters patient well-being than Margie and Mrs. Cooper.

Jack: Also, her wholistic care shows how care and rights can work together. I think that arguing about care versus rights sidetracks us from a major struggle in health care. That battle is between those who believe that the moral sense is the essence of health care practice and those who think that health care practice is essentially application of instrumental reason. Our primary concern should be the place of morality in nursing and not theoretical squabbles predicated on the assumption that morality already has a major place.

Anne: The technocratic and bureaucratic tendencies in nursing obscure the moral sense of nursing. I'm concerned that faith in instrumental reason with its emphasis on efficiency is leading us away from the moral sense of nursing. What will happen to nursing when emphasis on efficient instrumental reasoning replaces concern for whole persons, for their rights, and for their well-being?

Jack: I am concerned about how personal relationships and rights will be incorporated into health care when it is interpreted as instrumental reason. It seems to me that, in such an interpretation, concern for personal relationships and for rights can only be tangentially incorporated into practice. Rights need to be integrally related to care. Remember, if Tom's rights had been respected, he would have died. What saved his life was Zaner's thoughtful caring presence that helped him find possibilities for a life worth living.

Anne: But we do need to recognize the place of rights in nursing care, but as an integral part of nursing care, not as an adjunct. Margie does that beautifully. She advocates Mrs. Cooper's rights through holistic and wholistic care.

Jack: I wish she had been able to articulate the moral worth of what she did more adequately. But that is a contribution to nursing that ethics should make.

Anne: I hope you philosophers recognize that ethics could not make that contribution without examples of moral excellence such as Margie's care for Mrs. Cooper.

Jack: If Margie's care of Mrs. Cooper didn't make me aware of it, Claire Hasting's holistic care surely would! Her sensitive response to her patient's suffering and her interpreting of that suffering as personal rather than merely professional is so obviously moral that it requires no elaboration.

Anne: She is able to relate to her patient personally in care that is practically and professionally excellent. That is the essence of holistic care. I am troubled whenever nursing is reduced to technical or professional efficiency supported by recognition of patient's rights and divorced from personal feelings and aspirations of particular patients. Claire and Margie show how holistic care can fulfill the moral sense of nursing and how wholistic care can foster holistic care.

Caring Presence: Midori and Beverly

Jack: The relationship of caring presence between Midori and Beverly is an exemplar of moral excellence. Beverly's way of telling the story discloses the moral worth of their relationship.

Anne: I'm amazed that Midori's caring presence for Beverly is what I first recall from the story.

Jack: The caring presence of Midori transforms Beverly's nursing care. Zaner often says that the caring presence of patients is beneficial to the caregiver. He believes that this aspect of caring is much neglected.

Anne: He puts it more strongly than that. He emphasizes that caring itself is beneficial to the caregiver. Remember how Beverly affirmed that caring for Midori made her realize what it really means to be a nurse.

Jack: That's true, but care giving for some patients is not rewarding for nurses. In our study of fulfillment in nursing, most of the least fulfilling situations for nurses concerned patients who were uncooperative and unappreciative (Bishop & Scudder, 1990).

Anne: That's why caring for patients like Midori is so fulfilling for nurses. When "Midori moments" occur, nursing makes sense and is worthwhile. New possibilities of care are envisioned and a deeper quality of care is evoked.

Jack: But we have been so captivated by Midori that we have neglected Beverly. I think it's because we expect caring presence from nurses but not patients, especially when they are in pain and facing imminent death.

Anne: Isn't a good nurse one who sensitively responds to the caring presence of a person like Midori? One reason we so remember Midori in this story is that Beverly's sensitive description of her makes us aware of what a magnificent person Midori is. In addition, Beverly's response to Midori is so subtle and unobtrusive that its quality is easily unrecognized.

Jack: Talk about engrossment! Listen to this. "Her breathing was shallow and rapid. With each labored breath, her neck muscles strained and her abdomen protruded. We looked at each other, searching for the right thing to say. Only our tears came. Then silence." (See page 61.)

Anne: I want nursing students to read that. They need to learn when to be silent. They feel they must help and that talking helps, but often silence helps.

Jack: But silence helps more in a relationship of co-presence. I am struck by how Beverly and Midori are continually present to each other in speech, in silence, in touch.

Anne: Such deep relationships of co-presence cannot be created. They can only be evoked and anticipated. Knowing how to help someone through trying times without intruding and imposing is excellent nursing. Unfortunately, such caring presence is underappreciated as nursing excellence in this day of intervention.

Jack: Why in the world do nurses label as *intervention* everything they do to, for, and with patients? Would it make an ounce of sense to say anywhere in this story that Beverly intervened in the life of Midori? The one who is changed the most by their relationship is Beverly.

Anne: Well, before I met you, I used interventionist language and never really thought about it. It makes sense to talk about intervening in the life history of a disease. I know that interventions leading to cure have improved health care. But labeling personal relationships as interventions makes no sense. Such usage is especially inappropriate during a time when nurses are trying to rid themselves of the medical model.

Jack: In my naiveté, I always thought that the disease intervened in the life of the patient. Further, I believe that good health is the primary goal of health *care*. Cure contributes to health care, and I suppose intervention language makes sense in that context.

Anne: But Midori is beyond cure. She needs care and she is cared for sensitively, personally, and compassionately by Beverly. I feel that Midori would have made it all right without Beverly, but Beverly's caring presence helped her greatly. As Midori said, "These last two days have been the most important days of my life. I am grateful that you have helped me through them." (See page 62.) Helping someone through trying times without intruding or imposing is excellent nursing, but it also is an example of ethical care in nursing practice.

Jack: Caring presence assures you that you really matter. That's why it is important to understand the place of caring presence in affirming a person's worth. We philosophers attempt to establish worth by arguments that assign persons to a status or place them in a category, but a real felt sense that affirms your worth comes from experiencing caring presence.

Anne: Until now, I've never thought of intimate hands-on care as a way of affirming the worth of a person. But I've always thought that intimate relationships are at the heart of nursing. Others must feel the same way because the ethical in nursing is so often identified with caring presence.

CALLED TO CARE

Jack: I am sure that I'm not called to care in the tactile, intimate way that you nurses are.

Anne: Your caring usually involves thinking. I've learned from you that I can care by thinking. We nurses seem to dissociate thinking about meaning from caring. We do believe that instrumental reasoning is necessary in many nursing functions, such as formulating a plan of care. But we don't think enough about the meaning of nursing care, and we don't realize that one way to care about nursing is to think about it. Also, we don't recognize that thinking with patients about the meaning of proposed treatment and care is caring for them.

Jack: The tendency to think of thought as abstract and divorced from concrete and practical affairs is not limited to nurses. It is a general tendency in our culture. James challenged this misconception by asserting that the good life comes from being concretely and practically called by visions of a better life. He rejected both idealistic visions of the good life divorced from practical reality and so-called "realistic" approaches to life that eliminated visions of the good. He believed that we are called to care by people actually making demands on us and by seeing possibilities for a better life in the events in which we are involved.

Anne: In the parable of the Good Samaritan, the Samaritan is called to care by the plight of the injured man. The Samaritan's compassionate response is an example of what Noddings calls natural caring. It also discloses the meaning of holistic care in that the meaning of neighborly care, the call to care, compassionate care, and actual nursing care are all integrally related to each other.

Jack: It is a powerful disclosure of the moral imperative of responding to the call to care with nursing care. I was dismayed at the subtitle the editor of the *Journal of Christian Nursing* gave to an article we wrote, "On Being a Neighbor" (Bishop & Scudder, 1997). In spite of the fact that we interpreted the story of the Good Samaritan as a call to care, the editor subtitled the article—without our approval—"Nursing's Moral Standard." In so doing, she misdirected our readers by indicating that we were following traditional morality in seeking a moral standard by which to measure the goodness of nursing care. Approaching ethics as responding to a call to care is very different from using moral standards to measure moral goodness.

Anne: I'm always uneasy about using religious material in a book addressed to a general audience because it can so easily be misinterpreted. For example, I wonder if our omission of the religious context of the Good Samaritan will disturb the faithful? However, I would think that the faithful would be more concerned about our failure to treat religious ethics in our book. For many nurses, moral commitment involves religious faith.

Jack: I am glad you put it that way. I believe, as did my professor of Christian ethics, that an ethics should stand on its own without requiring religious faith. He did insist, however, that the religious implication of the ethics be considered.

Anne: Surely you are not proposing that we treat the religious implications of our nursing ethics in the conclusion of our book.

Jack: No, but I can indicate how a religious person might interpret our nursing ethics. God calls the faithful to care for those in need, regardless of religious affiliation. In current theological language, this call is spoken of as "ministering to the world" to distinguish it from ministry to a particular religious group.

Anne: The Good Samaritan ministered to the world. He did not ask if the injured man was a fellow Samaritan before he responded to his plight with compassionate nursing care.

Jack: Being called by God to minister to the world can readily incorporate our nursing ethics into the Jewish and Christian faiths—and others as well—even though our ethics can and does stand on its own.

Anne: Pellegrino's interpretation of profession can also speak to those who profess a religious faith and to those who do not. For Pellegrino, the meaning of being a professional is professing to use skill and knowledge to care for the well-being of clients. That profession is a moral imperative for all professionals. Those who are religious could interpret it as being called by God to minister to the world.

Jack: Does Pellegrino's interpretation of profession mean that nurses are not professionals if they merely enter nursing as a job and are proficient in the knowledge and skills of nursing?

Anne: I can answer that from my own experience. I don't believe that I entered nursing as a call to care. I was very much like Lashley who initially entered nursing as a job—not as a calling. Like Lashley, I was called to care by engaging in the practice of nursing with its inherent moral sense. I have come to believe that nurses are continually called to care for particular patients in different situations by their plight and the moral sense inherent in nursing care. Most nurses do act from a call to care. They just don't recognize or articulate their care in that way.

Jack: Philosophers could help nurses recognize and articulate the moral sense of nursing.

Anne: I not only want nurses to recognize the moral sense of their practice, but to respond to that recognition with good patient care. Such themes as the meaning of being a good nurse, holistic and wholistic care, caring presence, called to care, and ethics of practice are drawn from nursing practice and address moral concerns as practicing nurses encounter them. These themes may not be considered *real* ethics in some philosophical circles, but I believe that exploring these themes is valuable to nurses who are attempting to fulfill the moral sense of nursing practice.

Jack: Ethical considerations can issue calls to care, but not as forcefully as concrete examples. Patients like Midori would call into caring even a nurse with a narrow technical and professional view of nursing, and Beverly's response to Midori would call nurses into sensitive and deep relationships of caring co-presence.

Anne: Exemplars can forcefully call us into moral actions and relationships. But doesn't the call to care need to be rooted in an interpretation of the meaning of being human?

Jack: Werner Marx (1992) attempts such a move by saying that all humans face mortality and all humans need compassionate love from each other. Although I believe he is right on both counts, I am disturbed by his rooting ethics of compassion in human needs rather than in recognizing the moral worth of human compassion and of fellow human beings.

Anne: I've noticed that you often speak of roots rather than foundations. Is that because you want to remain rooted in the Greek and Judeo-Christian traditions without being committed to the foundational approach?

Jack: In a certain sense that's true, but I took the term *roots* from Heidegger (1962). Some of his students used to say that Heidegger had roots instead of toes. Seriously, the term *roots* is appropriate for Heidegger's interpretation of human being as being-in-time. Heidegger was challenging modern rationalism that grew out of the Greek contention that the world was founded on *logos*, an atemporal rational order that was eternal. In contending that we were beings-in-time, Heidegger was rejecting traditional logos thinking. We did that when we eliminated *the* good nurse from the second chapter and instead treated being a good nurse as fulfilling the moral sense of nursing that has grown out of an ongoing nursing tradition of fostering human well-being.

Anne: That moral sense does call us to care. I'm glad we got rid of the earlier title for Chapter 2, "*The* Good Nurse."

Jack: "*The* good nurse" sounds like we're seeking Plato's ideal form of "*the* nurse." Unfortunately, the reaction against this form of idealism has been so strong that it obscures the value of trying to grasp the meaning of being good. Taylor (1991) is right when he says that being authentic is vacuous if it means no more than being able to choose autonomously this or that course of action without some claim to be fostering moral good. Speaking of being a good nurse—either in the sense of being an excellent practitioner or a morally good person—makes no sense without understanding the meaning of and commitment to being a good nurse.

Anne: When we talk of the moral sense, almost immediately people challenge us by saying, "How do we know what the moral sense is in this day of cultural relativity and ethnicity?"

Jack: We can't absolutely know in this post-modern era in which our traditional foundations have been cut out from under us. However, I find Taylor (1991) informative when he says that striving to be authentic makes no sense apart from being able to make significant moral judgments. Likewise, nursing as practiced makes no sense apart from its moral sense.

Anne: If this book has helped nurses recognize the moral sense and become committed to it, I will be satisfied. However, I don't believe that will satisfy those critics who keep pressing us for *the* foundation of nursing ethics.

Jack: Nor will it satisfy those nurses who say it doesn't make sense to talk about the moral sense in a time when we are confused about foundations. Yet, they continue to make moral judgments in their practice, judgments that presuppose that nursing has a moral sense. Benner, Chinn, Gilligan, Noddings, Zaner, Marx, Taylor, Pellegrino, and James issue a call to care that does not require traditional foundations.

An Ethics of Practice

Anne: Because nursing has a moral sense that is inherent and primary, it makes sense to talk about an ethics of practice. The moral sense of nursing means fostering the well-being of clients, and that also is the meaning of practice.

Jack: We need to distinguish ethical activity required in practice from general nursing practice, however. Fostering the well-being of the client with a shot of penicillin is different from doing it by ethical considerations.

Anne: But nurses work in both ways and, as we have said, both are integrally related to each other.

Jack: They can, however, be distinguished from each other. For example, you tell me that it is necessary to turn persons in the right way so that they won't get bed sores. That doesn't strike me as an ethical activity, even though by doing it correctly you are fostering the patient's well-being.

Anne: I thought that we just wrote a whole book trying to help nurses see how their everyday practice involves ethical considerations, not just resolving the big moral questions that usually are treated in traditional nursing ethics books.

Jack: We did. But let me try to further clarify the distinction between ethical considerations in practice and general practice by considering the case of Tom, even though it's a medical case. Questions such as whether a dialysis machine can make Tom's continued living possible, how long he can live on dialysis, how often he will have to have dialysis concern medical practice. But considering what will make Tom's life worth living under the conditions imposed by dialysis, given all of Tom's other problems, strikes me as ethical considerations in practice. That's what Zaner gets Tom to consider (pp. 168–173).

Anne: Almost any nurse could have helped Tom consider the implications of dialysis for his life project.
Jack: Of course. When nurses or physicians help patients understand how medical or nursing care relates to their life plans or projects, nurses and physicians are engaged in ethical considerations.
Anne: So when Tom's physicians are prescribing and giving dialysis, they are fostering the moral sense of health care. But they are doing so by engaging in medical practice, not ethics.
Jack: Yes! I believe I am competent to engage in health care ethics, but it's inconceivable that I could engage in medical or nursing practice. If I did engage in ethical considerations with nurses concerning their care, then these ethical considerations would be a *part of* nursing care rather than *apart from* care.
Anne: Let's examine some examples of ethical considerations that are *a part of* nursing care rather than *apart from* it. In the previous chapter, all of the examples disclose the meaning of an ethics of practice—Tom, Lara, Barbara's patient, and Mr. Jones.
Jack: Recall how Mary helped Mr. Jones learn to relive the body that he was so alienated from and of which he was so afraid. Mr. Jones seemed like an entirely different person when he returned to the unit and swept up his nurse and hugged her. He fulfilled the role of one-cared for, as Noddings interprets it, both in expressing his appreciation for care given and by demonstrating his engagement in the human project of living well in the world. Mary became his advocate both by helping him determine the meaning of his illness and treatment for his life and by helping persuade his physicians to turn off the machine and try another form of therapy.
Anne: We nurses have talked so much about advocacy that most nurses will readily understand that being a patient's advocate means engaging in ethics in practice. But I believe that nursing ethics includes more than advocacy, as it is usually understood in nursing. For example, Mary is engaging in ethics by reminding Mr. Jones of his wife's faithful support. Directing him to his relationship with his wife helps him realize that continuing their relationship makes undergoing painful therapy worth it. This is similar to Zaner's helping Tom recognize the value of his work, which led Tom to undergo dialysis. Both cases concerned helping patients discover what makes painful and trying treatment worth enduring.
Jack: But Lara did not have the option of undergoing difficult treatment that would save her life. She had so much to live for and so little time. Her nurses engaged in ethics by helping her live as well as possible during her final days.
Anne: Barbara's patient faced a different problem. He had lost everything that made his life worth living. Barbara engaged in ethics by getting down on his level and befriending him.

Jack: I think that we have made our case for an ethics of practice, but we need to further clarify the meaning of ethics in practice. We can do so by describing a way of viewing the relationship of ethics and practice that is quite different from ours. This approach to ethics assumes that practice is primarily concerned with technology and science. In this practice, when physicians and nurses encounter moral problems, they call in the expert—an ethicist—to solve the moral problems.

Anne: This implies that medical and nursing care is one thing while ethics is another. Practice creates moral problems, and outsiders—usually educated in philosophy or theology—are brought in to solve problems raised in medical or nursing care. But don't those who hold this position believe that the ethical problems are related to care?

Jack: They do recognize that ethics is related to care, but that relationship is usually an adjunct one rather than a holistic one. For example, a physician limits medical care to restoring the efficient functioning of the body understood as an anatomical machine. Even though this physician regards a human being as a body and the body as a machine, he/she could rightfully claim that prescribing a drug, performing an operation, or hooking the body up to a machine is fulfilling the moral sense of health care by fostering the patient's well-being.

Anne: Few nurses would reduce the patient's well-being to the efficient functioning of the body understood as a machine. We care for the whole person, not just an efficiently functioning anatomical machine.

Jack: Let's further consider the implications for health care of caring for the whole person by examining another hypothetical example from medicine. A physician who believes that the anatomical body and the person are one decides that a basketball player needs an operation to ensure the efficient functioning of her body. This operation will prevent her from playing pro basketball. The basketball player says, "No way!" The physician complains that his patient doesn't know what's good for her and calls in an ethicist.

Anne: The physician is calling in the ethicist to rid himself of a nuisance question that is not, for him, involved in care. For him the issue is clear: the patient ought to have the surgery because it will improve the functioning of the body. But if we care for the whole person, we should relate her care to her life project. Frankly, I've never read anything in nursing literature that does not assume that consideration of life project, values, and moral commitment are not integral aspects of nursing care.

Jack: If nursing care is concerned with life projects and nursing ethics is concerned with how these projects relate to the nursing care given, then ethical considerations are integral and necessary aspects of nursing care.

Anne: Ethical considerations are as important for the patient as they are for the nurse. The physicians and the ethicist, in their consideration of what to do with the patient who did not want to take lithium because he enjoyed the mania high, did not help the patient face the moral meaning of his decision. They were only concerned with whether to treat or not treat.

Jack: The patient ought to have been given an opportunity to consider whether his decision was morally right rather than having the ethicist or the physicians make this decision for him. Thus, considering what is morally right is integrally involved in informing consent. Put differently, we believe that nurses are responsible for helping patients face the moral meaning of their patients' choices regarding illness and treatment.

Anne: But some patients, such as Midori, do not appear to need help in making moral decisions. She seems morally sensitive to her choices concerning her illness and its treatment. She decides not to undergo surgery that would probably kill her even though she prefers dying under anesthesia to dying by suffocation. She is willing to die of suffocation in order to live the rest of her life at home with her family. Beverly supports Midori in her struggle to reach that decision and empowers her to live with it and carry it out. Beverly's care supports her patient's life project—a life project that seems personally, morally, and medically sound.

Concluding Dialogue

Jack: We have been developing an ethics of practice that includes the meaning of being a good nurse, the relationship of ethics to wholistic and holistic care, caring as a moral calling and as caring presence, and ethics as an integral aspect of nursing care.

Anne: Nursing has an inherent moral sense and this moral sense is concretely instantiated in the practice of nursing care. Being a morally good nurse requires concern for the well-being of the patient that is expressed in effective, attentive, and skillful nursing care. Nursing care is experienced by both nurse and patient as caring presence, and this experience is beneficial for both and confirms the worth and humanity of each.

Jack: Ethical considerations are involved in nursing because nurses are concerned with how the life project of each patient will be affected by illness and treatment. These considerations concern the relationship of the lived body to self, others, and world.

Anne: Only recently have we nurses begun to think about the meaning of nursing. During my professional life, thought in nursing has primarily concerned how to do this or that, research modeled after science, and applying theories to practice. I hope that our book will call nurses to thoughtful care. I believe that nursing ethics should evoke thinking about concrete practice in ways that help nurses, individually and collectively, to fulfill the moral sense of nursing.

Jack: Our reflexive dialogue has explored how ethical consideration can contribute to understanding and fulfilling the moral sense of nursing. Nursing ethics helps nurses determine whether their practice, individually and collectively, lives up to its moral sense and whether that moral sense is adequate for the challenge of today's world. It also helps nurses recognize and be open to relationships of caring presence that affirm the humanity of patients and support them in their efforts to live well. In addition, ethics helps nurses to hear and answer calls to care given through the moral sense of practice, compassion for others, passion for authentic being, and new possibilities for well-being in nursing practice. Finally, it helps nurses engage in care that includes whole persons, their relationship to the world, and their personal life projects.

STUDY QUESTIONS

General Questions Concerning the Theme of the Book

1. Review Anne and Jack's brief summary of the major themes and the purpose of this book. Which of these themes spoke most forcefully to you as a future or present practicing nurse? Why? What themes did they fail to include that you would have included? Why?
2. Why did Anne and Jack entitle the book "Nursing Ethics: Holistic Caring Practice?" Do you believe that this title describes the content and purpose of the book? Why or why not?
3. How do Jack and Anne justify their approach to ethics in the beginning pages of the reflexive dialogue? After having read the book, do you think that their approach to ethics makes sense?

Questions Concerning the Reflexive Dialogue about the Relationship of Ethics and Practice

1. Gadow's interpretation of nursing as existential advocacy is one of the major moral interpretations of nursing. Why do Anne and Jack believe that Margie is an excellent existential advocate for Mrs. Cooper? Do you agree with their contention that her practice extends the meaning of Gadow's interpretation of existential advocacy? Why or why not?
2. One of the major discoveries of philosophers and others in the last half of the 20th century was how language structures our way-of-being in the world. Do you agree with Anne's contention that Margie's state-

ments about the meaning of her nursing care for Mrs. Cooper indicate that she does not fully grasp the meaning of advocacy or the moral sense of nursing? Why or why not? Do you believe that nurses often fail to grasp the moral significance of their care because of inadequate linguistic expression? If so, how can study of ethics help nurses express the moral worth of their practice in language?

3. Why does Jack criticize the use of most intervention language in nursing care? Do you agree or disagree with him? Why? Give an example of an inappropriate use of intervention language in nursing that obscures its moral sense. What language more appropriately describes the moral sense of what was called an "intervention"?
4. One of the major conflicts in nursing ethics is between those who focus ethics on patient rights and those who focus ethics on care. Do you believe that Jack is correct in describing Margie as a forceful advocate of the moral imperative of nursing? That Anne is correct in describing Margie's care as skillfully maneuvering through a web of connection to persuade others to join her in fulfilling the moral sense of nursing? Why?
5. Why is Jack perplexed over the conflicts between advocates of rights and of care? Do you agree with him? Why or why not?
6. What does Jack believe is the primary struggle in nursing ethics? Do you agree with him? If not, what do you believe the primary struggle is?
7. One issue raised in ethics is whether ethics is merely thinking about what it means to be moral or whether it includes evoking moral goodness. What does the dialogue concerning Beverly and Midori indicate that Anne and Jack believe about the role of ethics in nursing practice? Do you agree or disagree with them? Why or why not?
8. Anne and Jack contend that thinking can be a way of caring for patients and for the practice of nursing. Does holistic nursing require such care? Give examples from the book or from your own experience that support their contention. Do you agree or disagree with their assertion that thinking about the meaning of nursing practice is much neglected in contemporary nursing? Why?
9. Why would nurses who practice holistic care believe that nurses have a moral obligation to help patients consider the moral import of their care and treatment?
10. How does interpreting ethics as responding to a call to care differ from traditional ethics? What do James, Marx, and Taylor contribute to this approach to ethics?

REFERENCES

Bishop, Anne H., & Scudder, John R. Jr. (1990). *The practical, moral, and personal sense of nursing*: A *phenomenological philosophy of practice*. Albany, NY: State University of New York Press.

Bishop, Anne H., & Scudder, John R. Jr. (1997). On being a neighbor: Nursing's moral standard. *Journal of Christian Nursing* 14(4): p. 9–12.

Gadow, Sally. (1980). Existential advocacy: Philosophical foundation of nursing. In S. F. Spicker & S. Gadow (Eds.), *Nursing: Images and ideals*. New York: Springer.

Heidegger, Martin. (1962). *Being and time*. (J. Macquarrie & E. Robinson, Trans.) New York: Harper and Row.

Marx, Werner. (1992).*Toward a phenomenological ethics: Ethos and the life-world*. Albany, NY: State University of New York Press.

Ricoeur, Paul. (1977). Phenomenology and the social sciences. In M. Korenbaum (Ed.), *The annals of phenomenological sociology* II (pp. 145–149). Dayton, OH: Wright State University.

Taylor, C. (1991). *The ethics of authenticity*. Cambridge, MA.: Harvard University Press.

APPENDIX

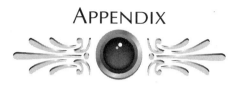

NURSING ETHICS

Sara T. Fry

The development of nursing ethics has paralleled the development of nursing as a profession. As nursing has evolved from the use of rules of hygiene in the care of the sick (Nightingale, 1859) to a profession that defines its practice realm as the promotion of health, prevention of illness, restoration of health, and the alleviation of suffering (International Council of Nurses [ICN], 1973), so has nursing ethics evolved from following rules of conduct in attending the sick (Robb, 1921) to an identified field of inquiry within bioethics (Veatch and Fry, 1987).

EARLY INTERPRETATIONS OF NURSING ETHICS

Early interpretations of nursing ethics tend to be associated with the image of the nurse as a chaste, good woman in Christian service to others and as an obedient, dutiful servant. Florence Nightingale's good nurse was committed to the ideal of doing what was right and had responded to a religious calling to nursing. Being of the highest character, she was disciplined by moral training and could be relied upon to do her Christian duty in service to others.

This view of the good nurse as a good woman pervaded early textbooks on nursing ethics. In addition to being physically and morally strong, Isabel

---

Reprinted from *Encyclopedia of Bioethics* revised edition by Warren Thomas Reich, editor. Volume 4. Macmillan Library Reference USA, Simon & Schuster Macmillan, 1995. © Warren T. Reich. Reprinted by permission of The Gale Group.

Hampton Robb thought that the nurse must be a dignified, cultured, courteous, well-educated, and reserved woman of good breeding. Like Nightingale, she considered the nurse's work as ministry, "... a consecrated service, performed in the Spirit of Christ..." (Robb, 1921, p. 38). Thus, moral virtue, moral duty, and service to others were established as important foundations upon which later interpretations of nursing ethics would be built.

At first, nursing ethics as practiced was virtually indistinguishable from nursing etiquette and the performance of duty. Nursing etiquette included forms of polite behavior such as neatness, punctuality, courtesy, and quiet attendance to the physician. The nurse demonstrated her acceptance of her moral duties by following rules of etiquette and by being loyal and obedient to the physician (Robb, 1921). Early textbooks on the subject describe nursing ethics as the ideals, customs, and habits associated with the general characteristics of a nurse and as doing one's duty with skill and moral perfection.

Some important distinctions were made between etiquette and ethics. Nurses learned proper ward etiquette in order to promote professional harmony in patient care; such etiquette became the foundation for all other nursing behaviors. Ethics, however, was taught to promote moral excellence and technical competence on the part of the nurse. Ethics was viewed as a science, the knowledge of which would enable the nurse to carry out prescribed duties with moral skill and technical perfection.

Following World War II, the nurse's role in patient care slowly shifted from that of the physician's obedient helper to that of an independent practitioner, held accountable for what had been done or not done in providing patient care. A shift in the understanding of nursing ethics accompanied this shift in roles. The nurse's moral responsibilities were no longer couched solely in terms of obedience to authority and institutional loyalty. Rather than someone who carried out the decisions made by others, the nurse now claimed authority for independent clinical decisions in patient care, including ethical decisions.

Contemporary nursing ethics began to develop in several directions. First, recently developed codes of nursing ethics were revised. Second, dramatic changes occurred in the teaching of nursing ethics. Third, nurses' attitudes, values, moral development, moral-reasoning abilities, and ethical practice or behavior were empirically studied. Fourth, the moral concepts of nursing practice were philosophically analyzed. Fifth, consideration was given to the development of theories of nursing ethics.

THE DEVELOPMENT AND REVISION OF NURSING CODES OF ETHICS

As professional nursing developed, nursing organizations discussed the need for a code of ethics for nursing practice. In the United States, the 1897 meeting of the newly constituted American Nurses' Association (ANA) was the first occasion for members of the profession to discuss a possible code of ethics for nursing. The ANA House of Delegates, however, did not accept a code of ethics until 1950. Revised in 1960, 1968, and 1976, the ANA Code for Nurses has served as a model for the development of nursing codes of ethics in other countries. Revised in 1985, the "interpretative statements" of the ANA Code delineate ethical principles that prescribe and justify nursing actions in the United States (ANA, 1985).

While the development of the ANA Code for Nurses was in process, the ICN, established in 1900, was developing an international code of ethics. A draft of an international code of nursing ethics was presented at the 1953 ICN Congress held in Sao Paulo, Brazil. The ICN Congress accepted the Code for Nurses and had it translated into several languages. The Code for Nurses was revised in 1965 and 1973 and reconfirmed in 1989. The ICN published guidelines on the use of the Code for Nurses in 1977 (ICN, 1973).

A significant number of national nurses' associations throughout the world have developed codes of ethics (Sawyer, 1989). Among the areas of agreement in nursing codes of ethics are nursing responsibility for practice competence; the need for good relations with co-workers; respect for the life and dignity of the patient; protection of patient confidentiality; and the nurse's ethical responsibility not to discriminate against patients on the basis of race, religious beliefs, cultural practices, or economic status (Sawyer, 1989). Like other professional codes of ethics, nursing codes provide important ethical standards that nurses can refer to when faced with questions of ethics or unethical practices on the part of co-workers and institutions. They are also an important historical record of the ethical concepts and principles considered important to nursing practice over time. Their periodic revisions have helped to shape the development of modern nursing ethics.

Codes of professional ethics are always hard to enforce. In the United States, the ANA Committee on Ethics encourages implementation of the elements of the Code for Nurses by supporting ethics education in nursing programs and by distributing copies of the Code for Nurses to nursing students. The ANA Committee on Ethics has also developed model policies and procedures that state nurses' associations can adopt in the processing of alleged violations of the Code for Nurses (Committee on Ethics, 1980).

Like all professional codes of ethics, nursing codes are hard to apply to patient-care situations. Since their statements represent moral ideals rather than specific action guides, professional nursing organizations have developed lengthy interpretations of nursing codes of ethics, or produced guidebooks with case applications of a code (Fry, 1994). In the United Kingdom, the Central Council for Nursing has published advisory documents to supplement its Code of Professional Conduct (United Kingdom Central Council, 1989).

Teaching Ethics in Nursing Education

During the 1970s, models for nurses' ethical decision making taught in nursing education programs were critically examined. A study of ethics teaching in 209 accredited baccalaureate nursing programs in the United States revealed that general ethics content was integrated into the curricula of two-thirds of the programs surveyed (Aroskar, 1977). The majority of the programs also expressed a need for the teaching of more specific nursing ethics content. Several textbooks on nursing ethics helped define this content (Benjamin and Curtis, 1986; Davis and Aroskar, 1991; Jameton, 1984; Veatch and Fry, 1987). According to these textbooks, both the teaching of ethics in nursing curricula and the analysis of ethical conflicts as they occur in nursing practice could enhance nurses' ethical decision-making abilities. They also agreed that the ethical problems nurses most often experience involve balancing harms and benefits in patient care, protecting patients' autonomy, and distributing nursing-care resources.

As various approaches to teaching ethics in nursing education developed, a consensus emerged that the overall goal of teaching ethics to nurses is to produce an ethically accountable practitioner who is skilled in ethical decision making. Intermediate goals of ethics teaching are to (1) examine personal commitments and values in relation to the care of patients; (2) engage in ethical reflection; (3) develop skill in moral reasoning and moral judgment; and (4) develop the ability to use ethics for reflection on broader issues having policy implications and for research on the moral foundations of practice. These goals focus on the fact that ethics is a form of inquiry that is used by every nurse in clinical practice. Broad general acceptance of these goals in nursing education prompted research into nurses' ethical decisions and the types of ethical issues nurses confront in patient care.

Nursing Ethics Research

The earliest record of a nursing ethics research project was Rose Helene Vaughan's 1935 study of the diaries of ninety-five student and graduate nurses who recorded the ethical problems they encountered in nursing practice over a three-month period. Vaughan's analysis identified 2,265 moral problems, 67 problems of etiquette, and 110 questions about ethical behavior. The ethical problem the nurses faced most often was the lack of cooperation between nurses and physicians and among nurses in general. Other ethical problems noted were: duties to the nursing school, lying (including dishonest charting), duties to patients, lust, and problems of temperance. Vaughan concluded that the problem of lack of cooperation her subjects experienced signaled nurses' growing awareness of their responsibilities to society and the role they were playing in patient care. She recommended more emphasis on ethics education in nursing to ensure a high standard of individual morality, which she believed would "raise the nursing professional above and beyond the slightest suggestion of social disapproval. . . ." (Vaughan, 1935, p. 105).

Despite this early interest in nurses' ethical problems, nursing ethics research did not begin in earnest until the 1980s. Research efforts initially focused on the ethical reasoning abilities and ethical behaviors and judgments among practicing nurses (Ketefian and Ormond, 1988). These studies focused on the ability of the nurse to make moral judgments, the hypothetical ethical behavior of the nurse, and nurses' perceptions of ethical problems. Methodologically, the studies were designed to document empirically the cognitive abilities of nurses to make moral judgments.

A few studies in nursing ethics have measured nurses' ethical decision-making styles, factors influencing nurses' ethical decisions, and the consistency of the way nurses make ethical decisions (Ketefian and Ormond, 1988). Nursing ethics research has also turned to the study of the attitudes and values of nurses concerning ethical issues (Davis and Slater, 1989), ethical conflicts nurses experience in the care of patient populations with severely disabling conditions (Norberg, Asplund, and Waxman, 1987) and those receiving long-term tube feedings (Wilson, 1992). The use of nursing-care resources by do-not-resuscitate (DNR) patients in intensive-care units as well as the impact of the DNR order on nursing interventions has been the subject of another study (Lewandowski, Daly, Modish, Juknialis, and Youngner, 1985). Still another study has identified variables that are the best predictors of a DNR classification and the extent of nursing care required by the DNR patient (Tittle, Moody, and Becker, 1991).

During the 1980s and early 1990s, the focus of nursing ethics research shifted from the study of nurses' ethical perceptions and behaviors, and of how nursing ethics was taught to the study of how nurses make ethical decisions and plan patient care when confronted with complex moral issues. Certain areas, however, remain unexplored. For example, the particular role of nurses in ethical decisions that affect patients is not very clear. Nurses' abilities to recognize moral values, make ethical decisions, and support patients' or family members' decisions are believed to be very important to the quality of patient care. However, little is known about the types of ethical decisions made by nurses and how they affect patient outcomes.

Another area that should be more carefully evaluated is the theoretical frameworks used to interpret study results in nursing ethics research. Since nursing is largely practiced by women, theoretical structures should include the process of ethical decision making by women as well as by men. Furthermore, researchers should use structures that can account for the nature and process of ethical decisions made by nurses in contrast to those of other health-care workers, such as physicians (Fry, 1989). This means that theoretical structures that are developed from the study of one gender alone or that consider ethical decisions as decisions made by physicians might not be appropriate for the study of nurses' ethical decisions. In considering appropriate theoretical frameworks, clarity about the moral concepts of nursing is very important.

MORAL CONCEPTS OF NURSING ETHICS

Advocacy, accountability, collaboration, and caring are moral concepts that comprise the foundation for nurses' principled, ethical decision making (Fry, 1994). They are important because they enjoy a firm place in nursing standards and ethical statements throughout the history of the nursing profession and help define the ethical dimensions of the nurse-patient relationship.

Advocacy. Advocacy may be defined as the active support of an important cause (Fry, 1994). In nursing, it describes the nature of the nurse-patient relationship and has been interpreted as a legal metaphor for the nurse's role in relation to a patient's human and moral rights within the health-care system (Winslow, 1984). Others have interpreted advocacy as the ideal expressed when individuals are assisted by nursing in the exercise of self-determination (Gadow, 1980), or the moral concept that defines how nurses view their responsibilities to the patient (Lumpp, 1979).

Advocacy is said to be associated with courage (Winslow, 1984) and heroism (Lanara, 1981). It may also be understood as the means by which the nurse participates with the patient in determining the meaning that the experience of illness, suffering, or dying has for that individual (Gadow, 1980). Lumpp (1979) has even argued that two general, ethical principles—fidelity and respect for human dignity—are rooted in the advocacy concept. Some nurse ethicists have interpreted advocacy as the ethical principle that underwrites what nurses do to protect the human dignity, privacy, choice (when applicable), and well-being of the patient (Fry, 1994). This last view of advocacy seems most consistent with the values expressed in nursing codes of ethics and the primary ethical responsibilities of the nurse.

Accountability. The concept of accountability seems to have two major attributes: answerability and responsibility (Fry, 1994). Nurses are assumed to carry personal responsibility for nursing practice and are expected to justify or "give an account" of their nursing judgments and actions according to the profession's ethical standards or norms. Terms of legal accountability for nursing practice are contained in licensing procedures and state-regulated nursing practice acts, while terms of moral accountability appear as norms in codes of nursing ethics and other standards of nursing practice. By virtue of agreeing to perform nursing care, the nurse accepts accountability for performing such care according to these standards and norms.

Accountability is said to be a basic moral value in nursing practice (Fry, 1994) and a moral foundation for nursing practice (Yarling and McElmurry, 1986). A few codes of nursing ethics have focused on accountability as a central moral concept (ANA, 1985; United Kingdom Central Council, 1984), and at least one national nursing organization has provided documentation on the extent of nursing accountability in professional practice (United Kingdom Central Council, 1989).

Cooperation. Cooperation is active participation with others to obtain quality care for patients, collaboration in designing nursing care, and reciprocity to those with whom nurses professionally identify. It implies consideration for the values and goals of those with whom one works. The concept of cooperation encourages nurses to work with others toward shared goals, make mutual concerns a priority, and sacrifice personal interests to maintain the professional relationship over time.

Cooperation has been included in many codes of nursing ethics as a moral concept of nursing practice (Canadian Nurses' Association, 1989; ICN, 1973; New Zealand Nurses' Association, 1988). While early views on nursing ethics linked cooperation to a special loyalty shared by members of the professional group (Robb, 1921), later views linked cooperation to the need to compromise individual goals and interests in order to achieve a mutually determined and higher level of patient care (Benjamin and Curtis, 1986; Fry, 1994).

Caring. The moral concept of caring has long been valued in the nurse-patient relationship. Caring behavior is considered essential to the nursing role and is presumed to affect how humans experience health as well as life itself. Nurse caring is directed toward the protection of the health and welfare of patients and indicates a commitment to the protection of human dignity and the preservation of human health (Fry, 1994).

Recent feminist interpretations of human caring relate caring to the protection, welfare, or maintenance of another person (Noddings, 1984). Others have defined caring as a moral obligation or duty among health professionals (Pellegrino, 1985), and as a form of involvement with others that engenders concern for how they experience their world (Benner and Wrubel, 1989). These views indicate two attributes of the concept. First, caring is a natural, human sentiment and is the way all humans relate to their world and to each other (Noddings, 1984). It exists as a structural feature of human growth and development before caring behaviors actually commence. Second, caring is linked to moral or social ideals such as the human need to be protected from the elements or the need for love. Caring, in this sense, might be interpreted as a special duty that exists between individuals and an ethical obligation within a given context.

The concept of caring has been identified as an important moral foundation for a nursing ethic that protects and enhances the dignity of patients. Caring is said to be a moral art central to health-care practices (Benner and Wrubel, 1989); the moral foundation for the nurse-patient relationship (Huggins and Scalzi, 1988); and a moral virtue of nursing practices (Knowlden, 1990).

Theories of Nursing Ethics

Progress in the development of a theory of nursing ethics has been slow, partly because of the disputes about the relationship of nursing ethics to medical ethics and to the discipline of ethics itself. Some ethicists claim that there is little that is morally unique to nursing practice (Veatch, 1981). The same moral issues confront everyone in the health-care setting, regardless of whether one is a physician, nurse, or patient. This means that nursing ethics is a legitimate term only insofar as it refers to a subcategory of medical ethics. Since medical ethics is the ethics of all judgments made within the biomedical sciences, nursing ethics is simply the ethical analysis of those judgments made by nurses in much the same way that physician ethics is the ethical analysis of those judgments made by physicians. Any theory of nursing ethics will, therefore, be exactly like medical ethics theory. According to this view, a theory of nursing ethics may not even be necessary.

Others argue that nursing ethics is not just another form of applied ethics, especially medical ethics (Jameton, 1984). If the moral concepts and obligations inherent in nursing practice are different from (yet compatible with) those of other health professions, then nursing ethics may have a distinct voice in health care. If so, nursing ethics will use traditional and contemporary forms of philosophical analysis to describe the moral phenomena of nursing practices, to critically assess the language and conceptual foundations of nursing practice, and to raise normative claims about the aims of nursing practice within the health-care sphere. It will provide a perspective on what is good and bad, right and wrong in nursing practice and propose ethical principles to guide nursing judgments and actions. It will be nursing ethics theory and not medical ethics theory.

Regardless of its form, any theory of nursing ethics will need to address the relevance of the moral concepts of nursing practice in the years ahead. As the twenty-first century reveals new moral challenges in health care, nursing ethics must respond with conviction about the integrity of its moral concepts and methods of ethics teaching. If it is to claim its promise as a form of philosophical inquiry for the field of bioethics, it must also continue to move ahead on the expansion of nursing ethics research and the development of practice-based theories of nursing ethics.

References

American Nurses' Association (ANA). 1985. *Code for nurses with interpretative statements.* Kansas City, MO: Author.

American Nurses' Association (ANA) Committee on Ethics. 1980. *Guidelines for implementing the code for the nurses.* Kansas City, MO: Author.

Aroskar, Mila. A. (1977). Ethics in the nursing curriculum. *Nursing Outlook* 25 264.

Benjamin, Martin, & Curtis, Joy. (1986). *Ethics in nursing*. (2nd ed.). New York: Oxford University Press.

Benner, Patricia E., & Wrubel, Judith. (1989). *The primacy of caring: Stress and coping in health and illness*. Menlo Park, CA: Addison-Wesley.

Canadian Nurses Association (CNA). (1989). *Code of ethics for nursing*. Ottawa: Author.

Davis, Anne J., & Aroskar, Mila A. (1991). *Ethical dilemmas and nursing practice*. (3rd ed.). Norwalk, CT: Appleton and Lange.

Davis, Anne J., & Slater, Patricia V. (1989). U.S. and Australian nurses' attitudes and beliefs about the good death. *Image*, 21(1), 34–39.

Fry, Sara T. (1989). Toward a theory of nursing ethics. *Advances in Nursing Science*, 11 (4), 9–22.

Fry, Sara T. (1994). *Ethics in nursing practice: A guide to ethical decision making*. Geneva: International Council of Nurses.

Gadow, Sally. (1980). Existential advocacy: Philosophical foundations of nursing. In S. F. Spicker and S. Gadow (Eds.), *Nursing: Images and ideals* (pp. 79–101), New York: Springer.

Huggins, Elizabeth A., & Scalzi, Cynthia C. (1988). Limitations and alternatives: Ethical practice theory in nursing. *Advances in Nursing Science* 10 (4), 43–47.

International Council of Nurses (ICN). (1973). *Code for nurses: Ethical concepts applied to nursing*. Geneva, Switzerland: Author.

Jameton, Andrew. (1984). *Nursing practice: The ethical issues*. Englewood Cliffs, NJ: Prentice-Hall.

Ketefian, Shake, & Ormond, Ingrid. (1988). *Moral reasoning and ethical practice in nursing: An integrative review*. New York: National League for Nursing.

Knowlden, Virginia. (1990). The virtue of caring in nursing. In M. M. Leininger (Ed.), *Ethical and moral dimensions of care* (pp. 89–94). Detroit, MI: Wayne State University Press.

Lanara, Vassiliki A. (1981). *Heroism as a nursing value: A philosophical perspective*. Athens: Sisterhood Evniki.

Lewandowski, Wendy, Daly, Barbara, Moclish, Donna K., Juknialis, Barbara W., & Youngner, Stuart J. (1985). Treatment and care of 'do-not-resuscitate' patients in a medical intensive-care unit. *Heart and Lung* 14 (2), 175–181.

Lumpp, Francesca. (1979). The role of the nurse in the bioethical decision-making process. *Nursing Clinics of North America* 14 (1), 13–21.

New Zealand Nurses' Association Professional Services Committee. (1988). *Code of Ethics*. Wellington, New Zealand: Author.

Nightingale, Florence. (1859). *Notes on nursing: What it is, and what it is not*. London: Harrison and Sons.

Noddings, Nel. (1984). *Caring: A feminine approach to ethics and moral education*. Berkeley: University of California Press.

Norberg, Astrid, Asplund, Kenneth, & Waxman, Howard. (1987). Withdrawing feeding and withholding artificial nutrition from severely demented patients: Interviews with caregivers. *Western Journal of Nursing Research* 9 (3), 348–356.

Pellegrino, Edmund D. (1985). The caring ethic: The relation of physician to patient. In A. H. Bishop & J. R. Scudder (Eds.), *Caring and coping: Nurse, physician, patient relationships* (pp. 8–30). Tuscaloosa, AL: University of Alabama Press.

Robb, Isabel Hampton. (1921). *Nursing ethics: For hospital and private use.* Cleveland, OH: E. C. Koeckert.

Sawyer, Linda M. (1989). Nursing codes of ethics: An international comparison. *International Nursing Review* 36 (5), 145–148.

Tittle, Mary Beth, Moody, Linda, & Becker, Mark P. (1991). Preliminary development of two predictive models for DNR patients in intensive care. *Image* 23 (3), 140–144.

United Kingdom Central Council for Nursing, Midwifery, and Health Visiting. (1984). *Code of professional conduct for the nurse, midwife, and health visitor* (2nd ed.), London: Author.

United Kingdom Central Council for Nursing, Midwifery, and Health Visiting. (1989). *Exercising accountability: A framework to assist nurses, midwives, and health visitors to consider ethical aspects of professional practice.* London: Author.

Vaughan, Rose Helene. (1935). The actual incidence of moral problems in nursing: A preliminary study in empirical ethics (Doctoral dissertation, Catholic University of America, Washington, DC).

Veatch, Robert M. .(1981). Nursing ethics, physician ethics, and medical ethics. *Law, Medicine, and Health Care* 9 (5), 17–19.

Veatch, Robert M., & Fry, Sara T. (1987). *Case studies in nursing ethics.* Philadelphia: J. B. Lippincott.

Wilson, Donna M. (1992). Ethical concerns in a long-term tube feeding study. *Image* 24 (3), 195–199.

Winslow, Gerald R. (1984). From loyalty to advocacy: New metaphor for nursing. *Hastings Center Report* 14 (3), 32–40.

Yarling, Roland R., & McElmurry, Beverly J. (1986). The moral foundation of nursing. *Advances in Nursing Science* 8 (2), 63–73.

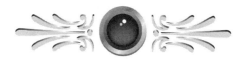

INDEX

Accountability, 127, 128
Advocacy, 76–77, 108, 127, 128
Agape, 25
American Medical Association (AMA), 79
American Nurses Association (ANA), 124, 125, 128
Aroskar, Mila A., 125–126
Asplund, Kenneth, 127
Authenticity/authentic care
   call to, 75–82
   and competency, 24, 25
   and empowerment, 20
   Heidegger, Martin, 48
Autonomy
   dialogue on, 5, 6, 11
   and posture, 95–96
   and wholistic care, 33, 34, 109

Ball, Barbara L., 59
Becker, Mark P., 127
Being Called to Care (Lashley, Neal, Slunt, and Hultgren), 69
Being-in-time, 115
Benjamin, Martin, 125–126, 129
Benner, Patricia, 10, 116
   caring, 129
   competency, 23
   good nursing, 21–22
   intuitive judgment, 25
   co-presence, 60–61
   clinical ethics, 94, 99
Berman, Louise M., 69
Bioethics, 123, 130
Bishop, Anne H., 1, 2, 3
   calls to care, 72, 75, 76, 78, 80, 112–116
   caring presence, 47, 111–112
   clinical ethics, 86
   concluding dialogue, 119–120
   dialogical interpretation, 4–14
   good nursing, 106–107
   nursing practice, 116–119
   reflexive dialogue, 105–106
   wholistic and holistic care, 33, 107–110
Body, lived, 55–57
Buber, Martin, 10, 43–48, 62, 104
Bureaucracy, 11–12
Business ethics, 8

Calls to care, 67–69
   authenticity, 75–82
   compassion, 73–75, 81–82
   concrete, 71–72
   dialogue on, 112–116
   neighbor's plight, 72–73
   "of course" response, 69
   profession, 70–71
Canadian Nurses' Association, 128
Caring, 48–54, 127, 129. *See also* Calls to care; Ethical caring; Holistic care; Natural caring; Wholistic care
Caring presence, 41–43
   caring, 48–54
   dialogue on, 111–112
   personal relationships, 43–48
   presence, 55–63
Carpenito, Linda J., 80
Central Council for Nursing. *See* United Kingdom Central Council
Chinn, Peggy, 67–68, 104, 116
Christian ethics, 113–114, 123. *See also* Good Samaritan
Clinical ethics, 85–86
   in holistic care, 98–100
   requirements for, 86–98
Code for Nurses (ANA), 124–125
Code of Ethics (AMA), 79
Code of Professional Conduct (United Kingdom Central Council), 125

Collaboration. *See* Cooperation
Committee on Ethics (ANA), 125
Compassion, 72–75, 81–82, 115
Competency, 23–24
Concern, 53, 54
Concrete calling, 71–72
Context of Self, The (Zaner), 55
Cooper, Debra, 29–32, 49, 103, 107–110
Cooperation, 33, 34, 127, 128–129
Co-presence, 55, 60–63, 111–112, 115
Cousins, Norman, 38, 42
Cucci, Mary, 96–98, 99–100, 104, 106, 117
Cultural relativity, 115
Curtis, Joy, 125–126, 129

Daly, Barbara, 127
Davis, Anne J., 125–126, 127
Decision-making. *See* Moral decisions; Moral dilemmas; Moral judgments
Dependent care, 48
Desires, conflicting, 51–52
Diekelmann, Nancy, 54
Do-not-resuscitate (DNR) patients, 127
Dreyfus, Hubert L., 25
Dreyfus, Stuart E., 25
Duty, 123
Dyck, Beverly, 62, 104, 111, 115, 119

Education, ethics in, 125–126
Empowerment, 20, 52–53
Encyclopedia of Bioethics (Fry), 3
Engelhardt, Tristram, 36
Engrossment, 48, 53, 54
Ethical caring, 49–51, 53
Ethical codes, 79, 124–125
Ethicists, 2, 91, 118–119
Ethics of Authenticity, The (Taylor), 81
Ethics of compassion. *See* Compassion
Ethnicity, 115
Etiquette, 123–124
Existential advocacy, 76–77, 108

Feminist ethics, 109
Foundations, 115, 116
Frankl, Viktor, 38
Freedom, 60
Fry, Sara T., 3
  bioethics, 123
  call of profession, 70
  codes of ethics, 125
  moral concepts of nursing ethics, 127, 128, 129
  research, 127
  teaching ethics, 125–126

Gadamer, Hans George, 10, 25
Gadow, Sally, 46, 76, 108, 128
Gilligan, Carol, 10–11, 33–34, 42, 109, 116
God, 114
"Good nurse, the" 26, 115
Good nursing, 17–26, 103, 105, 106–107
Good Samaritan, 72–73, 81, 104, 113–114

Harder, Ingegerd, 18–19, 47
Hastings, Claire, 35–37, 103, 110
Health care reform, 34–35
Heidegger, Martin, 10, 48, 53, 76, 115
Heron, Echo, 51
Holistic care, 29–33, 35–38
  clinical ethics in, 98–100
  dialogue on, 107–110
Holocaust, 38
Huggins, Elizabeth A., 129
Hultgren, Francine H., 69

Identity, 77
I-It relationships, 43–46
I-It (Thou) relationships, 46–47
In-between stance, 32–33
Informed consent, 7–8
Informing consent, 7–8
Instrumental reason, 79, 110, 112–113
Integral care, 67–68
International Council of Nurses (ICN), 123, 124–125, 128
Intervention, 80, 112
I-Thou relationships, 43–46, 47, 48, 62

James, William, 10, 71–72, 104, 116
Jameton, Andrew, 125–126, 130
Jesus, 72–73
Jewish faith, 114
Journal of Holistic Nursing, 107
Judeo-Christian tradition, 73–74, 113–114, 115, 123
Juknialis, Barbara W., 127

Kantian autonomy, 5, 6
Ketefian, Shake, 126, 127
Knowlden, Virginia, 129
Kohák, Erazim, 54
Kramer, Robin, 92–94
Kreiger, Delores, 42
Kwant, Remy, 53–54

Lanara, Vassiliki A., 128
Language, 108, 109, 112, 114, 130
Lashley, Mary Ellen, 69, 104, 114
Lewandowski, Wendy, 127

Life projects, 118, 119
Lived body, 55–57
Logos, 115
Lumpp, Francesca, 128

Marx, Werner, 10, 73–75, 104, 115, 116
McElmurry, Beverly J., 128
Messner, Roberta, 41
Mickunas, Algis, 46
Modish, Donna K., 127
Moody, Linda, 127
Moral concepts, of nursing ethics, 127–129
Moral decisions, 33–34, 126, 127
Moral desires, conflicting, 51–52
Moral dilemmas, 7, 51–52
Moral judgments, 24, 116, 126
Moral problem, 7
Moral turpitude, 78
Mortality, 74, 115
Motivational shift, 48, 53, 54
Moyers, Bill, 52

Natural caring, 49–51, 53
Neal, Maggie T., 69
Neighbor, meaning of, 72–73
New Zealand Nurses' Association, 128–129
Nightingale, Florence, 123
Noddings, Nel, 10, 104, 116
 caring presence, 43, 48–54, 55, 61, 117
 calls to care, 69, 76, 82
 moral concepts of nursing ethics, 129
Norberg, Astrid, 127
Nursing education, ethics in, 125–126
Nursing ethics
 early interpretations of, 123–124
 moral concepts of, 127–129
 research, 126–127
 teaching, 125–126
 theories of, 129–130
Nursing etiquette, 123–124
Nursing practice
 caring in, 52–54
 dialogue on, 116–119
 integral nature of, 19–21
 and nursing ethics theories, 130
Nussbaum, Martha, 52

"Of course" response, 69
Orem, Dorothea, 76
Ormond, Ingrid, 126, 127

Pain, 11
Pellegrino, Edmund, 70–71, 79, 104, 114, 116, 129
Perry, Clifton B., 6
Personal care, 17–26
Personal relationships, 43–48
Phenomenology, 106
Phronesis, 25
Plato, 115
Pleasure, 11, 77
Potency, 60
Practical wisdom, 25–26
Practice. See Nursing practice
Presence, 55
 co-presence, 55, 60–63, 111–112, 115
 dialogue on, 111–112
 reflexive, 55–57
 vivid, 55, 57–60
Profession, call of, 70–71

Quinn, Janet, 42

Rationalism, 115
Rawlinson, Mary, 36
Reason, instrumental, 79, 110, 112–113
Reciprocity, 48
Reflexive dialogue, 105–106
Reflexive presence, 55–57
Reform. See Health care reform
Reich, Warren Thomas, 123
Relationships. See Personal relationships
Relativity, cultural, 115
Religious faith, 113–114
Research, 126–127
Responsiveness, 48
Rew, Lynn, 107
Ricoeur, Paul, 10, 106
Rights, 109, 110
Robb, Isabel Hampton, 123, 124, 129
Roots, 115

Scalzi, Cynthia C., 129
Scudder, John R., Jr., 1, 2, 3
 calls to care, 72, 75, 76, 78, 80, 112–116
 caring presence, 46, 47, 48, 111–112
 clinical ethics, 86
 concluding dialogue, 119–120
 dialogical interpretation, 4–14
 good nursing, 106–107
 nursing practice, 116–119
 reflexive dialogue, 105–106
 wholistic and holistic care, 33, 107–110
Slater, Patricia V., 127
Slunt, Emily Todd, 69

Smith, Huston, 37
Smith, Margie, 29–32, 49, 103, 106, 107–110
Spiritual meaning, 37–38

Taylor, Charles, 10, 75–81, 82, 104, 115, 116
Teaching, ethics, 125–126
Technology, 11–12, 79–80
Theories, of nursing ethics, 129–130
Thinking. See Instrumental reason
Tillich, Paul, 38
Time, limited, 51–52
Tittle, Mary Beth, 127
Tolstoy, Leo, 71
Toombs, Kay, 95, 98–99
Traditionalists, 11
Triadic dialogue, 47–48
Troubled voices: Stories of Ethics and Illness (Zaner), 87

United Kingdom Central Council, 125, 128
Utilitarianism, 5, 6

Vaughan, Rose Helene, 126
Veatch, Robert M., 123, 125–126, 129
Vivid presence, 55, 57–60

Waxman, Howard, 127
Web of connection, 34
We-relationships, 60
Wholistic care, 11, 29, 33–34, 107–110
Wilson, Donna M., 127
Winslow, Gerald R., 128
Wisdom, practical, 25–26
Wrubel, Judith, 23, 94, 129

Yarling, Roland R., 128
Youngner, Stuart J., 127

Zaner, Richard, 10, 116
  caring presence, 41, 42, 43, 55–63, 104
  clinical ethics, 4, 85–98